Chemoland

What to expect when you were not expecting
chemotherapy for breast cancer

By Tamzen Whelan

DEDICATION

To all the women whom have gone before me, and to the ones
that must follow. There are way too many of us.

AUTHOR'S NOTE

We are all individuals, and no two people will experience chemotherapy in the same way. However, there are some common threads that tie us together; facing chemotherapy is frightening at best, it will take its toll in varying degrees physically, emotionally and mentally, but we will get through it. I began this book during my radiation phase of treatment with the hopes of offering practical tips while it was all still fresh, and an emotional connection for anyone about to undergo treatment, including caregivers. We are not in this alone.

Part One
My Story

Chapter 1
Join the Fight

*"I know God won't give me anything I can't handle.
I just wish he didn't trust me so much."*
— Mother Teresa

"Welcome to the club," the nurse said, handing me a pink, plastic band.

Her mouth twisted upward into a smile, but there was only pity in her eyes. Or maybe it was embarrassment.

"Thanks…?" I muttered, certain that I would never slip that thing onto my wrist. I didn't sign up for this, and I wasn't going to commemorate it by wearing a rubber bracelet that announced my disease.

I fingered the obtrusive object and eyed the trash can in the corner. I wanted to chuck it in there, but instead, shoved it to the bottom of my overstuffed bag where I knew I would never see it again.

I was actually very calm that day, unlike a lot of other days that had led up to it. I had just received the results from my biopsy, confirming what I already knew; I had cancer. But I never thought hearing the words "you have breast cancer" would make me so happy, like I had just won a Pulitzer. I had convinced myself over the past month and three days that I had lymphoma and was going to die soon, so finding out that it I had breast cancer was the best news ever. Nonetheless, I was 46 and the first person in my family to ever have pre-menopausal cancer of any sort, and I wanted that thing out of me, whatever it was. It was growing, and I couldn't understand why it was still in me.

"Cancer doesn't grow that fast," I had been told.

"We want to get all of our ducks in line," was another explanation.

My gynecologist had found a lump in my left breast during a routine exam. I had gone in because I had some spotting in-between cycles, and he felt what he thought was a cyst. He was sending me for a trans vaginal ultrasound because of the spotting, and decided to get me a bilateral breast ultrasound as well, just to be safe. Both came back negative, but several cysts were found in my left breast, so it was decided that I should have a diagnostic mammogram, again, just to be safe. That was on July 19, 2013.

On July 29, I had the mammogram, immediately followed by another ultrasound, both showing a lump under my right arm measuring 1.5 centimeters. How was that possible? It hadn't shown up at all just 10 days earlier!

"They must be looking at the lymph node," the technician had said while she maneuvered the cold wand around my breast.

Those words tortured me throughout the month of August. What I thought was going to be the biopsy wasn't scheduled until the 20th. A full three weeks knowing I had this foreign growth in my body. When the day finally arrived, I showed up at the doctor's office early after driving 45 minutes to get there only to find out that my appointment had been cancelled due to an emergency surgery. I was happy to know that the surgeon did emergency surgeries in case I needed one, which I was convinced that I did, but then I was informed that my appointment wasn't even for a biopsy after all! It was for a consultation. I didn't need to discuss this lump, I needed it taken out, or at the very least to find out what it was. My new appointment was scheduled for two days later.

My anxiety was growing, and my heart rate was accelerating with each day that passed. On Thursday morning, I got another dreaded call telling me that my appointment again had been cancelled. How could this be? The thing was now the size of a walnut, and I was having trouble shaving around it. It grew more every day, and I feared the worst.

"You may as well order me an autopsy, rather than I biopsy!" I sobbed into the phone.

"Sorry," was all she could offer.

She was only the messenger after all.

I paced the house, then the yard, and then the neighborhood, working myself up into a full grown panic attack. Then I shook myself off, put my anxiety aside and picked up the phone. I was determined to find a new surgeon that would be able to see me that day. One of my first calls was to the Robert and Carol Wiseman Cancer Center, a place I would later consider my second home. I told the very nice woman on the other end of the line my predicament. She said that she knew of a surgeon who might take me within the next couple of days, but that first we should push to see the one that had already been assigned to me. She also told me that he was one of the best, and was in high demand. That made me feel somewhat better, but what good were highly capable hands if it were too late? I got off the phone with her, and she promised to act as my advocate and get a straight answer about my ever changing appointments.

A short two hours later, I received a phone call from the surgeon's office letting me know that my appointment was miraculously back on. That woman was a Godsend. Later, I would meet her in person and be able to thank her.

"I can't give you the biopsy today," the doctor informed me at my consultation later that day, and I saw the look of concern on his tight face.

A new appointment was set for the following Tuesday. He would come in just to see me. I knew then that it was bad.

I did not sleep for those five nights, waiting. The lump was now the size of an egg, and I was sure that I would be dead in a week.

During the day, I played movies that I did not watch. At night, I drank wine. Lots of it. I was completely unaware of the beautiful summer weather and the needs of my family, or anything else around me. If my teenage daughter had gotten pregnant and eloped, I wouldn't have noticed. The days were dark and time was a blur.

The day of the biopsy finally arrived, and I was a mess. An hour before I was supposed to leave, my insides began to hurt, and the room started to spin. I was sure that the cancer was now everywhere in my body, taking over. I doubled over in pain, and crawled to the front door like a wounded animal. I didn't want to be inside where no one could find me if I passed out. I managed to grab my car keys and phone on the way out, and collapsed on the front lawn. I was sweating from head to toe, and my body was like an icicle, cold and dripping all over. The pain was so intense that I could not move. I don't know how long I lay there, but not one person walked by, which was actually a blessing in disguise. Just when I was about to call 911, the phone rang.

"The doctor is early," the receptionist said. "Can you come in now?"

I told her I was in a lot of pain, and maybe needed to go to the ER instead.

"If you can drive, come to us," she said wisely. "You will see a doctor here."

Somehow, I made it to my car, ignoring the excruciating pain that clenched my gut, and fifteen minutes later, I waddled into the office. The nurse took a long look at me.

"We can't do the biopsy today," she said, "you are obviously in too much pain to sit still. We will have to reschedule for next Saturday," she informed me.

"NO!" I cried, wincing in agony, "strap me down if you must. I need the biopsy today!"

The doctor came in then, and took a few deep breaths. He had obviously been prepped on the situation.

"Have you been drinking?" he asked.

"What? No!" I answered.

"Not today, anyway," I added, thinking about all the wine I had consumed lately.

"Have you pooped today?" he probed with a straight face.

"Um, I'm not sure," I answered, "maybe not…"

"Well, we are doing the biopsy today," he informed me and the nurse after examining my stomach with his cold hands, "no matter what."

As soon as he plugged in the monitor and began inserting needles into my skin, the vice grip that had been twisting my insides all morning began to release, and I could feel the stress melt away. The ball had finally started rolling in the right direction. I realized then that the mind is so very powerful. It would take me many more lessons like this one before I would put that knowledge to good use.

I left there that day with a prescription for Xanax, and an appointment for seven days later to get the biopsy results. That week sailed by peacefully. I thought that there was nothing they could tell me that I didn't already know. I distantly feared chemo, and radiation, but all I could think about was getting that thing out of me.

"You will need radiation," he had said right before the nurse had given me the bracelet.

"No chemo?" I asked, feeling that those words were too good to be true.

"I don't think so," he answered, "unless I find something else during the surgery."

"Oh, thank God," I said vainly, "I just don't want to lose my hair!"

He eyed my long, golden pony tail which I had always considered to be my best physical asset, and ran his fingers through the loose strands.

"You do have beautiful hair," he said.

It was agreed that I would have a lumpectomy, rather than a mastectomy. He assured me that a lumpectomy followed by radiation had the same effectiveness as having a mastectomy. Before I left, he gave me a referral for a radiation oncologist, and I asked how soon I could have the surgery. The answer of one week satisfied me greatly.

"Ms. Whelan," the receptionist called to me as I was leaving the office.

"There is a problem with your insurance," she informed me when I turned back.

I spent the next week on hold with the insurance company. I was unable to get through to a person, and cursed repeatedly into the phone. How could this happen? Was it all the ultrasounds, and mammogram, and biopsy that had led to a reasonable conclusion of cancer and they had dropped me because of foreseen expense?

In-between calls of no avail to insurance, I spent calling the surgeon's office. Time was ticking away, and my alien lump was still growing strong.

"I would like to know my surgery date," I would say.

"The coordinator is very busy," I would hear, "but I'm sure she is working on it."

The calls to insurance got even worse. I was put on hold endlessly – up to two hours at a time without ever speaking to a person.

"I would like to know my surgery date," I would repeat the next day.

"We are working on getting a charity to sponsor you," I was informed.

I finally got an answer and I was livid. It was about money. They thought I couldn't pay without even asking me! Maybe it was the impression I had made on the day of my biopsy when I had stumbled into the office in my pajamas, covered in grass, after writhing in pain on my front lawn for an hour. Looking back, it was no wonder that the doctor had thought I was drunk. I had pretty much resembled the local bag lady. The next time I visited the office, I would be sure to be sporting my Coach handbag, and my grandmother's 2.5 carat diamond ring. I might even comb my hair – if I still had any.

That day on the phone, I had some not-so-nice words for them, and was grateful that the receptionist would not be the one to perform the surgery.

"Screw the charity!" I said in my new not-so-polite voice, "I need this thing out of me. NOW. Schedule the surgery, and I will pay for it!" I demanded.

Just when I needed one, another angel was sent to me in the form of my neighbor Bee. I had met her couple of months back at a BBQ. Our mutual friend now informed me that Bee was a pathologist at the same hospital that my surgeon was associated. I immediately got in touch with her, and it turned out that she knew the surgeon personally. She promised to go to his office as soon as we got off the phone and try to get a surgery date.

One hour later, the receptionist called to let me know that the lumpectomy had been scheduled for the following Wednesday, two weeks after I had received the biopsy results. Somehow, I would come up with the $10,000 within the next week.

Up until that time, I felt that there were two polar entities at play. And now, one of them was declared the winner. I just wasn't sure if good had really won out over evil. Perhaps there was someone upstairs looking out for me, and had managed to get the ball rolling in the nick of time. But maybe the cancer had already done the damage it needed to do, and so moving ahead with treatment would make no difference. Either way, the seas of resistance magically parted, and I finally got a real live person on the other end of the line at the insurance company.

"I'm sorry," she said, "it seems there was a clerical error. There is no problem with your insurance. It will be reinstated by the end of the day."

I refrained from speaking my mind in order to not ruffle any more feathers that might set things back. Now I had one less worry that I could scratch off of my growing list of concerns.

The lumpectomy itself was a breeze compared to the mental anguish I had gone through for the past month and a half. On September 18th, I arrived at noon after fasting since 10 p.m. the night before. I was immediately taken back to adorn my gown and get briefed by the attending nurse. I was asked a lot of questions concerning my anxiety, and given a pregnancy test. Once I was secured into my gurney and had my arm implanted with an IV which provided much needed fluids, my partner Jeff, was allowed to be by my side. He was the only one there since my family lived on the furthest side of the country from me, and my daughter was at school, which was how I wanted it.

She was 15 at the time, and I had decided that she would know everything from the beginning so that nothing would come as a shock. I had told her about the lump from day one, and the possibility that it could be cancer, and what that would mean. She was aware of all of my appointments, and I shared with her each piece of information as it came. However, I did spare her the details of my ongoing mental torment. That was not something she needed to know. I wanted her life to go on as normally as possible with minimal interruption. She played that role well throughout.

Jeff was able to stay with me for the next hour as they monitored my vital signs and we waited for the surgeon. Once he arrived, everything went quickly. I was injected with a dye that allowed for my lymph nodes to easily be seen, and it made me warm and tingly all over. Then I was dripped with a sedative that made me feel like I had had five margaritas. The last thing I remember is being wheeled into the surgery room where I was placed under a large head lamp. I was surrounded by white coats, and they were helping me onto a table. Then my lights went out. I woke up what seemed like five minutes later in the recovery room. I looked at the clock and was shocked to see that two hours had flown by. Upon inspecting my body, I discovered a plastic bulb strapped to my chest.

"Your drain," the nurse explained.

I would have to wear that thing for the next week, emptying it as it became full of the secretions from the surgery site. Lovely.

Jeff was then led into the room and he was all smiles.

"It's all good!" he said, almost giddy.

I had no idea what he was talking about. My head was still fuzzy from the anesthesia.

"No lymph nodes!" he clarified.

That *was* good news, and I had forgotten to worry about it.

I was in bed for the next few days, recovering from surgery, but I never needed to break into the pain medication that had been prescribed for me. Advil worked just fine. The mood around our house was one of elation: no cancer in the lymph nodes = no chemo = no hair loss. We were ecstatic! And I was surrounded by beautiful flowers that had arrived from friends and family from all over the country. I felt relieved, loved, and good. The nightmare was over.

NOT.

A week after the lumpectomy, I arrived early at my appointed post-op meeting with the surgeon.

"Everything looks good," he said as he removed the cumbersome drain that I had been wearing like an unwanted child strapped across my surgery site.

I became worried when he inspected my scar and frowned. There was a dimple where my breast tissue used to be.

"I will take care of that later," he said, as if I really cared about an indent in my breast at this point.

"You will need to see an oncologist," he continued, still inspecting his handiwork.

"You already gave me the referral," I said, happy that he was only worried about a minor crease where the alien cancer had been and was now gone.

"That was for radiation," he said looking up at me now, "you will need chemo."

Luckily, the walls didn't spin and the floor didn't open up and swallow me. I was in shock. His words were not real, and they bounced right off of me. I had had cancer. The lump was gone. There were no lymph nodes affected. I couldn't possibly need chemo.

"I need a second opinion, then," I said, somehow rationally.

"Trust me," he replied, "you can ask 50 doctors and 51 will tell you that you need chemo."

He went on to explain that the pathology report, which had been rendered by none other that my good neighbor B, had come back on my tumor which clarified that my cancer was "triple negative". Not estrogen receptor positive (ER+), not progesterone receptor positive (PR+), and not human receptor positive (HER2+). Negative for all three. In the case of hormone positive breast cancers, if the tumor is small enough, the patient will be given a hormone blocker in a pill form, such as Tamoxifen. This is usually prescribed for five years, and no chemo is necessary. Triple Negative breast cancer only accounts for around 15% of all breast cancers and is relatively unstudied. Therefore, no one as of yet knows what fuels it, making such targeted therapy an impossibility.

My head was now swimming because before that moment, I had no idea that there were even two different types of breast cancer. I thought breast cancer was breast cancer. I was about to get an education that I didn't want. Pretty soon I would be a walking oncological dictionary.

"And it is not in the earliest stage," he continued.

No shit, I refrained from saying. It wasn't really his fault that it had grown from 1.5 centimeters at the end of July to 2.5 centimeters by the time I had it taken out six weeks later. The official diagnosis was Triple Negative, High Grade (meaning it was fast growing), Invasive Ductal Carcinoma, Stage IIA. A mouthful. Little by little, I would investigate what it all meant.

"I would like you to meet another patient of mine," the doctor said. "She was diagnosed with the exact same cancer over a year ago."

He led me into his office, and a few minutes later a woman appeared. She had a full head of hair, but I couldn't stop staring at the braces she wore on both arms.

"From the neuropathy," she explained.

"The ner...what?" I asked.

"From the chemo. It made my hands go numb permanently. But

it is rare," she added after seeing my face go Gumby green.

I questioned the doctor's sanity for having me meet this woman.

"Do you have your port yet?" she asked.

Again, I had no clue what she was talking about. She pulled her blouse over to one side, revealing a small box that protruded from her chest just under the skin, like a microchip.

"It's where they infuse the chemo. Saves the veins," she explained.

"No," I said.

And I never will, I thought, but didn't say. There was no way I was going to exchange one alien in my body for another, especially not one that screamed PATIENT. It was bad enough that I was going to be bald. Unlike other diseases, being a victim of cancer offers no anonymity. With just one glance, the secret is out in the open for the world to see. In my mind, this meant being treated differently; looked at with curious pity rather than benevolent indifference. It also meant that I had to admit to myself the severity of what was happening to me. At the end of our meeting, the kind woman gave me her phone number, but we both knew I would never call.

"It is going to be a shitty year," the doctor said as I was leaving.

Year? He must have been exaggerating.

The most difficult part of that day was yet to come. I had to break the news to my family, and thus, shatter the fairytale ending that we had been living.

"How long will you be sick?" my daughter asked, probably thinking about all the dinners I wouldn't be able to cook her, and the rides I wouldn't be able to give her; what length of time she would be without a mother.

"I don't know," I answered truthfully because I really had no inkling.

"Weeks, months, or years?" she wanted to know, seeking some kind of gauge.

"Months," I guessed, knowing that she needed a concrete answer so that she could begin to process this new information.

The thought of it really being months terrified me. Could my family really get by without me for that long?

"Maybe I shouldn't do this," I said to Jeff later that night when we were alone.

"You are the quarterback in this," he said, giving me one of his adorable football analogies. "You make the calls. Whatever you decide, I will back you up."

He would be on my "team," but the decision was mine alone.

I spent the rest of the evening drinking wine, and sharing the news with my extended family. I never heard the words "don't do it."

Chapter 2
11:11

"The only thing we have to fear is fear itself."
— Franklin D. Roosevelt

About three years before my breast cancer diagnosis, I actually had premonitions of my own demise. I didn't think of it that way in the moment, but looking back, it is clear. At the time, I thought of it as more like visions. I was teaching English full time at the local community college in Albuquerque, and also writing my first book. I didn't have a lot of time to spend on the novel, and I would often visualize myself in a hospital bed with a laptop, scrambling to write to the end. I remember at that time how important it was that I be able to finish my book, and it seemed like death and the end of my book were competing. In my visions, I also had several notebooks. In those pages, I saw myself writing letters to my daughter and various family members.

Once we moved to Florida two years later, it went even further. I began giving my daughter advice on life, and driving tips in particular– just in case I wouldn't be around when she got her license. She was 15 at the time. I never thought anything was strange about this. In fact, I thought it was normal, and maybe it is; however, these visions and life lessons stopped sometime around the halfway point in my treatment.

Before cancer, I would have described myself as easygoing, extremely logical, and an optimistic realist. After cancer, I proved to be nervous, uptight, and shockingly superstitious. There was a lot that I didn't know about myself. Like the fact that I can be a drama queen, and that what I thought of as my superior analytical skills could morph into buying into worst case scenarios. Perhaps those traits were there all along, bubbling under the surface of a thin layer of security which now had exploded and lay in shreds before my eyes. I also learned that I fear death more than the average person. In fact, during that time, I completely altered my vocabulary. I would not utter one word that was associated with death. "I am dying of thirst," would carefully become "I would give anything for some water." I had never realized how many sayings there are in the English language that refer to dying, and how many I used on a regular basis: "I would kill to go to Hawaii," "you look like you are on your death bed," "don't kill yourself over it," "that cake is to die for." I would not even utter the words "this is the end" or "when it is over." And if anyone referred to my cancer in the present tense, I would quickly correct them.

"I HAD cancer," I would say.

And more typically, I would tell people, "I don't have cancer, I have chemo."

But more than the words, 11:11 was taking over my life.

I was in fact my own worst enemy. Every time I looked at the clock, whether it was am or pm, it read 11:11. In many eastern cultures, the number four is bad luck, and also associated with death. I thought it was a bad omen. At first, when it was approaching 11:00, I would just avoid looking at the clock until I thought enough time had gone by. But sometimes I couldn't resist peeking, so I started going for walks every day at 11 a.m., and made sure I was in bed by 11 p.m. When that became inconvenient, I plastered tape over all of the clocks in the house at 11 a.m. every day, remembering to unveil them before anyone else got home.

So I was greatly relieved that my first visit to the oncologist would be at 2:30 p.m. As usual, I arrived early, allowing plenty of time to work myself up into a frenzy. By the time the nurse called me, I had entered a full-blown panic attack. She took my blood pressure twice with the automatic cuff, and then moved on to the manual.

"Are you feeling OK?" she asked.

"What do you mean by 'OK'?" I replied.

"Well, like, are you going to have a heart attack?"

Not quite the right thing to say to someone having a panic attack. Against my better judgment, I looked at the screen. My blood pressure was 170/120. No wonder she was worried. She quickly left, and the doctor came in a few minutes later. I was pacing the four-foot by four-foot room when he entered.

"I'm having a panic attack," I informed him.

"Would you like me to come back in a few minutes?" he asked.

"NO!" I blurted. "I don't want to be alone!"

What I really wanted was a big bear hug, but I had just met the man, and besides, he didn't really strike me as the cuddly type.

"Well, then," he said, getting down to business, "your tumor was triple negative, and stage II, so you are going to need chemotherapy."

"Why!?" I asked a little too loudly for the small space, startling him. "If all of the cancer was taken out, and my lymph nodes are clean, why do I need chemo?"

I refused to call it chemo*therapy* because nothing about it seemed very therapeutic.

"Well," he said, clearing his throat, "if there is even one stray cell, the cancer will come back. Without chemotherapy, there is only an 80% chance that it won't recur."

"And with chemo?' I asked.

"88%."

I was going to have to think long and hard about this. Was chemo worth it for only eight percentage points?

"Add another four for radiation," he said, reading my thoughts.

We were now up to 92% chance of no more cancer, ever. But there was no way to tell if there was a stray cell or not. Chances were that I didn't need chemo at all. No one would ever know.

"How long will I be on chemo?" I asked, already feeling resigned.

"Five months," he stated.

I was stunned. My head dropped into my hands, and my long blonde hair swept the cold floor. I thought I was going to faint. The doctor grabbed my arm, and gently guided me backward into a chair. He then handed me three booklets on the specific chemo drugs he had already slated out for me, and I quickly scanned them, my eyes landing on the side effects.

"I don't think this is a good idea," I said.

One of the side effects that glared at me from the black and white page was "heart damage". I was down to 5 cigarettes a day since my diagnosis, but I had been a pack a day smoker for over 20 years. I voiced my concern, and he assured me that I would be having a MUGA, which stands for Multi Gated Acquisition scan (think huge EKG), to determine if my heart was indeed strong enough. This did not make my anxiety go down.

"But first you will need a port," he said.

"Huh uh. NO WAY!" I declared, picturing the alien in the woman's chest that I had met at the surgeon's office the week prior.

His eyes bulged to the point of popping, and he backed away from me toward the door.

"I'm going to send the nurse in," he said and made his escape.

The nurse arrived and explained to me why I needed a port.

"The chemo burns like acid, and you don't want it to get on your skin," she said.

If it burns like acid, I didn't want it going into my veins, either! I thought, and maybe should have said.

She took about five vials of blood from my arm, and sent me on my way.

One week later, despite all of my assertions, my port would be in place.

I left that day with a prescription for valium, an appointment for the MUGA and my port placement, and a time to return for my first dose of chemo, scheduled for two weeks later.

A bald woman was standing next to me as the receptionist handed me my paperwork. She leaned in closer, and I knew she wanted to offer me some words of advice, or encouragement, or maybe just empathy. I let my long blond hair slide over my face, making a thick curtain between us. I wasn't ready to be "one of them." A month later I would see this same woman in the elevator. She didn't recognize me with my beanie covering my matching bald head, but she greeted me like a sister.

"How are you feeling today?" she asked.

"Shitty," I replied and smiled.

"I wish I could shit," she said and we both chuckled.

The only other person in the elevator had gotten on at the radiation floor and had a full head of hair. We knew that there was no way that she could understand why we were laughing.

The day after I had my initial meeting with the oncologist my phone rang around 11 am. I picked it up, and the numbers 11:11 glared at me from the screen.

"Ms. Whelan?" the voice on the other end asked.

"Yes?" I answered.

"I'm calling from the oncology office. Your blood test indicates that your CEA markers are high, so the doctor wants to send you for a PET scan to determine if there is any cancer in your body, and if so where."

She was speaking a foreign language, but I did understand, "cancer in your body." She gave me my appointment time, and when I got off the phone, I ran to the bathroom and threw up. Was it really necessary to give me all those details?

The next day, the phone again rang around 11:00 a.m. I didn't answer it. I took a shower, paced the house, and finally looked at my phone. The call had come in at exactly 11:11. I didn't recognize the phone number, and I couldn't bring myself to listen to the message. I just could not face any more bad news. Finally, I decided to go somewhere friendly, and maybe listen to it there. I chose Barnes & Noble. Surely I would feel comforted being surrounded by all of those books. I methodically scanned the aisles, but it wasn't a book I was looking for. Instead, I was searching for a nice bald lady who might hold my hand while I listened to my voice mail, or better yet, listen to it herself and relay the message. No luck that day. Everyone there was wearing a full head of hair with the exception of a couple of older men, but they were a gamble. I leaned against the non-fiction rack, took out my phone, and held my breath while I bravely clicked on messages. It was the veterinarian reminding me of my dog's upcoming appointment. I slowly exhaled. I drove home with a stack of good reads, and a journal that I would write in faithfully over the course of my treatment.

When I was a teenager, I had a bad experience with pills. I had been given my first prescription drug - a simple muscle relaxant for severe menstrual cramps; I took two, and got in bed, hoping to feel "relaxed". However, twenty minutes later, my entire body felt weighed down, like I was under water. I tried to make it to the bathroom, but my limbs had turned to jelly, and left me in a heap, melting into the hardwood floor. It was hours before I recovered and was able to walk on my own. I have had several other similar experiences over the years, and finally learned that I am more sensitive to drugs than the average person. So unfortunately, I never put the Xanax or valium to good use like I should have. The only thing that calmed me was Jeff. When he offered to take the next week off to accompany me to all of those scary upcoming appointments, I didn't hesitate to take him up on it.

First stop was the MUGA.

The day started out with a mild panic attack, and Jeff took me to the beach to settle me down before my appointment. When we arrived at the hospital, I was feeling relatively calm, and was led into what looked like someone's very messy office; the only difference being the huge machine in the center of the room, where I was instructed to lie down. Then they injected me with something I am sure was radioactive and plugged me in. The machine started to flicker and buzz, and I started to freak out, sure that my heart was in such bad shape that it was making everything go haywire.

"Don't worry," the kind man said. "It's not you. This machine is just old."

Great. Then a tunnel slid around me, but there were windows on the side, so I could see out. A huge camera towered above me, and I was told that there would be two pictures, and each would take 10 minutes. I could feel the whoosh as my blood and heart beat did their thing, and kept repeating to myself that I was in the safest place possible if I were going to have a heart attack.

There were about five people in the room, and none of them were concerned with me whatsoever. The phone kept ringing, and they carried on with their paperwork. The camera clicked, and the second picture started. Finally, after what seemed like way longer than 20 minutes, it was over.

Five days later, I found myself back at the surgery center for the dreaded port placement. I was there for over three hours, but the actual procedure was quick and easy, lasting only 30 minutes. I was now officially a long-term patient. I didn't mind the port half as much as I had thought, but for the first couple of weeks, sleep was difficult because of surgeries on both sides of my chest.

Two days later I again arrived at the hospital for the PET scan. I thought I would take a valium for this, but there was no need. I hadn't slept a full night in over a month, and I was pretty much zonked out by the time the technician escorted me into a small room that was furnished with only a recliner. He injected me with my second radioactive dye of the week, and left me in the room alone for an hour. Jeff was just on the other side of the door, and it was comforting to know that I could call out to him if I needed. Instead, we held a texting conversation which helped the time pass.

Exactly one hour later, I was led into another room, with another machine. I lay on the table and the tube passed over me, quickly at first. I was fidgety with fear, and the tech had to keep reminding me to keep still. I wished I could. The machine slowed down, and then took five pictures, starting with my head. Each picture was supposed to take three minutes, but I am sure it was much longer. For the first couple of photos, I felt very claustrophobic, but once my head came out the other side of the tube, I relaxed. A little.

We ended that whirlwind of a week by prepping the house for my anticipated sick days. My computer was moved into the bedroom for easy access, we filled the cupboards with easy to grab snack food, and a friend made a much appreciated surprise delivery with enough frozen pasta dinners to last a month. I also ordered a dozen bandanas from Amazon, and several fancier head scarves, beanies and a cotton night cap from curediva.com. I was prepared, but would have to wait five whole days for the results of the MUGA and PET, which would also be The Big Day – CHEMO.

Chapter 3
The Perks of Chemo

"We are as happy as we make up our minds to be."
—Abraham Lincoln

Sunday night before The Big Day, my cell phone rang.

"Tamzen!" said the overly cheerful voice on the other end of the line.

It was my good friend Kim. We had met about a year and a half earlier when both of our families relocated to Florida. Jeff and her husband had landed their dream jobs at the same company. There were about eight of us women that would get together on a regular basis for morning coffee or evening wine. However, nine months after we made the move, the company folded, leaving all the families scrambling. At the time of my diagnosis, Kim and I were just about the only ones left in Florida. She had gone through breast cancer and chemo five years earlier, and was a great support and inspiration for me. About a month into my treatment, though, she would move away as well.

"I am calling to tell you the perks of chemo," she continued enthusiastically.

"OK," I said. "Let's hear it."

This was going to be good.

"You will have no hair. ANYWHERE!" she said.

"OK," I said, still doubtful.

"Just think about it. Your showers will be very quick, and you will save all that money on shampoo and razors," she explained.

"What else?" I asked.

"Your periods will be gone forever!" she said triumphantly.

That was a good one.

"Anything else?" I asked, getting in the mood.

"Well, no," she answered. "But in the end, you will be a much stronger person, more compassionate, and a lot more appreciative."

Those pearls of wisdom were lost on me at the moment. I had much more pertinent issues on my mind.

"But will I be able to drink wine, and go to the gym?" I asked.

"Some days, yes," she said. "You are not going to stop living."

Despite all those great things I had to look forward to, I still did not sleep that night.

Chapter 4
The Big Chair

"One is never afraid of the unknown; one is afraid of the known coming to an end."
— Jiddu Krishmamurti

I was not a good patient. My oncologist and the chemo nurses most likely would have given me a big frowny face instead of a bright shining star on my completion certificate if I had ever gotten one. On the first day of treatment, I paced the cramped interior of the hospital room waiting for the doctor, and the results. Jeff was perched on one of the two hard plastic chairs in the room, pinned in by the three over stuffed bags that I had brought with me: one with books and blankets, one with food and water, and the other with my laptop and journal. Finally, just when my blood vessels were about to burst, he walked in and nonchalantly announced that my heart was strong, and the PET scan showed no signs of cancer in my body. I let out a deep breath that I did not know I had been holding.

"Then why chemo?" I squeaked, hoping to get out of it while I still had my hair.

At this point, I had already done quite a bit of research on chemotherapy in general. The possible side effects terrified me, especially since I knew myself to be overly sensitive to drugs. Also, there was no guarantee that it would work. It is very possible to go through months of treatment, only to have the cancer come back despite it all. I had been looking for a way out, but the research also stated that triple negative breast cancer in particular can be highly susceptible to chemo. The doctor patiently explained to me again, that the tiniest of stray cells could cause the cancer to recur, and the PET scan could not necessarily detect that.

"Let's do it!" he said leading us out of the room as if we were headed to some greatly anticipated sporting event.

It would have been nice to have had a tour of the chemo room prior to this moment, but as it was, this was my first glimpse of it. There were big, brown recliners all lined up in a neat row. They almost looked comfortable. These were facing the large picture windows, where small stools were lined up for visitors. Jeff pointed out the great view of the Indian River, but all I could see were the bald heads rising above the backs of the chairs, and the poles next to each chair, dangling an assortment of IV bags that were plugged into each body somewhere below the head. I felt repulsed.

"Pick a seat," the chemo nurse said as we entered.

We chose a recliner in the far corner with the most privacy. Most of the patients had blankets pulled up over them due to the frigid temperature, and were asleep. I learned later that this was because a lot of the chemo drugs require a dose of Benadryl before administering in order to lessen the chance of an allergic reaction.

"This is IT," I said to Jeff as we took our places.

"There is no one Big Moment," he replied, reading my anxiety, "just a lot of little steps."

The first little step was for me to sign a form agreeing to take the chemo and acknowledging the side effects. If we hadn't been on the third floor, I might have jumped out the window in front of me.

The second step was for the nurse to draw blood to make sure that my white blood cell count was high enough to get treatment. At that time, I had no idea what a normal white blood cell count might be, but in the weeks to come, I would become quite intimate with my blood.

We waited for about a half an hour before we saw the nurse again, who came over to our far corner of the room to cheerfully let me know that my blood count was good. She instructed me to take one of the horse pills that had been prescribed to me for nausea, called Emend, and then she left. We had arrived that morning at 9:30. It was now 11:00 a.m.

Ten minutes later, the nurse came toward me again, now trailing four IV bags with long cords wrapped around her like snakes. I jumped from my seat and hurried past her to the restroom. There was absolutely no way I was going to allow her to plug me in at 11:11.

When I returned to my chair, it was safely 11:15, and the nurse was waiting. She first sprayed my port to numb it, and then inserted the needle. There was no pain, but it was disturbing. The first IV bag was what she called pre-meds. This included more anti-nausea medicine and steroids. I could see the clear liquid dripping down through the tube, and watched it until it hit my port. But even if I hadn't been watching I would have known that it had entered my body. I immediately began to feel jittery. It took about 30 minutes for the bag to empty its contents inside me at which time I was bouncing off the walls and might have done quite nicely if I were running a marathon. When the nurse came back the next time, she switched the IV line over to the bag holding what looked like red Kool-Aid.

"Are you ready for your first cocktail?" she asked smiling.

I thought she was trying to be funny, and maybe she was, but that is really what they call it. A personalized mixture of chemo drugs is a cocktail and adjusted according to your body mass. Like most breast cancer patients, mine consisted of Adriamycin – AKA the Red Devil, followed by Cytoxan, the combination of which is commonly referred to as A/C. I was slated to get this every other week for eight weeks, and then move on to Taxol, which would be once a week for 12 weeks.

"No," I said meekly, and Jeff took my hand.

Ready or not, it was coming down the line. I closed my eyes, and a few minutes later, knew for certain that the poison had reached my veins. Welcome to Chemoland. My arms and legs grew heavy and then began to tingle, and my head felt light. The nurse came back to check on me soon after because apparently, if an allergic reaction is going to happen, it occurs within the first 10 minutes. She was not alarmed by what I described to her.

"You will get through this," she said, and I began to relax.

Jeff and I spent the next hour munching on cheese and grapes and reading. I also guzzled three bottles of water because I had read that chemo can make you dehydrated, and water can also help flush out the toxins. Eventually, I had to go to the bathroom because of it. However, I would not go alone. With my port tied to the pole that held my chemo bags, I had to navigate with the entire contraption around the recliners, and hope not to trip. As I wheeled the evidence into the ladies room, it dawned on me then that I was now officially a cancer patient. There was no going back. I was one of them, and I was going to lose my hair. Then the bigger truth took hold; there is no "one of them" – cancer can blindside anyone, anywhere, anytime.

"Ms. Whelan?" the nurse called to me just as I was about to shut the door. "Don't be alarmed that your pee is pink," she said, "from the chemo."

Indeed it was.

Soon after, I was on to my third IV bag which held the Cytoxan, followed by a saline solution intended as a flush, and then we were done. All in all, it took five hours, and I was starving. I had read not to eat anything that you really enjoy as your first meal after chemo because you may develop a strong aversion to it forevermore. However, Jeff thought we should eat somewhere special, and I ended up with a huge lobster feast. Luckily, I still love lobster.

That night was rough. My legs felt heavy and tingly, I had a pounding headache, and I couldn't sleep. In fact, I got a total of two and a half hours, most likely due to the 20 milligrams of steroids that were pumped into me. In the morning, as instructed, I took another Emend for the nausea that I didn't have, accompanied by a steroid pill. Again, I began to feel jittery, but it was better than groggy.

That afternoon, I went back to the doctor's office for a white blood cell booster called Neulasta. The nurse warned me that I may experience some bone pain. That would be like an analyst forecasting 9/11 as a minor inconvenience to the US. Instead, it was the wrong kind of gift that kept on giving. Two hours later, every inch of my body was in agony. It felt like my bones were immersed in a raging inferno, and there was no way to put out the flames which finally extinguished on their own around midnight. Another sleepless night.

The week passed much like this: after taking the Amend and steroid in the mornings, I would fly around the house in a cleaning frenzy, but take a head-long crash in the afternoon as the steroid wore off. I drank no less than 12 bottles of water per day, and I did not sleep at night. By Thursday, I could add heart palpitations and extreme dizziness to the list, to the point that I could not walk. Just getting to the bathroom was a chore.

Some women actually go to work while they are on chemo, so I knew it was not going well for me. I began to make a list of side effects. Week One looked like this:

*Constipation (96 hours)
*Fatigue
*Heart Palpitations
*Extreme Dizziness (Off balance/ Can't walk)
*Tingling in limbs
*Head in a fog (Can't concentrate)
*Weight Loss (3 pounds)

The following Monday, I went back for blood work. Despite the Neulasta, my white blood cell count was low, a condition called Neutropenia. I was told to stay away from public places because if I caught any type of virus, my immune system would not be able to fight it off. That would be easy since I could barely get out of bed. When I told the nurse about my week one side effects, after insisting that heart palpitations and dizziness were not caused by chemo, she suggested that I see my cardiologist.

"I don't have a cardiologist!" I explained in frustration.

Before now, the most serious health issue I had ever had was a toothache.

By Wednesday of the second week after my first chemo I could function, and by Sunday I was feeling about 90% normal, except for the fact that thick tufts of my hair came out with my morning shower. It still flowed down to my waist, so I had my daughter cut it up to my shoulders, something she had begged me to do since she was in Kindergarten when her friend had cut all of her hair off. I figured I had nothing to lose if she gave me a Frankenstein cut because it would all be gone soon enough. She actually did a good job, and I got to experience what it was like to have short hair – luckily I liked it ok.

That evening the sea of depression engulfed me. What should have been a productive day instead left me washed up and in bed. I was feeling pretty much myself, but I knew that the next day I would have to get back on the Chemoland rollercoaster and face again all of the unknowns. I seriously questioned the sanity of that. However, bright and early Monday morning, I again found myself back in the doctor's office. Jeff came loaded with my chemo supplies, and I was armed with my list of side effects.

The constipation would be taken care of with Milk of Magnesia and a daily dose of over-the-counter Senokot-S. I was to try to counter fatigue by mild exercise, and limit rest to 45 minute intervals. To address the heart palpitations, I would no longer take the steroid pills which were slated as a possible cause. Having tingling limbs, my head in a fog, and weight loss, I would just have to deal with. However, when it came to my complaint of severe dizziness, and feeling off balance, he reiterated what the nurse had told me – that was not a side effect of chemo.

"We will keep an eye on it," he said, and sent me off to The Big Chair.

The chemo nurses followed the same routine as before. I hoped with all my heart that my white blood cell count would still be too low for treatment, but somehow it had bounced back over the week. Again I was given the steroid and anti-nausea drip, followed by Adriamycin, then Cytoxan, and then the flush. This time, though, I was out within three hours, and leaving behind me a trail of golden locks. That night I had Jeff buzz my hair down to an inch. When I looked in the mirror, I laughed, but I wanted to cry. What stared back was a freakish Chemoland version of me. The little hair that I had left was brown rather than golden blonde and significant patches were missing.

The following week was much like the first week but more intense. This was to be expected because chemo is cumulative. I slept off and on for a total of two hours on Monday night. Tuesday I went back for the Neulasta, and endured burning bones the rest of the day and night. There was no sleep to be had as my heart fluttered off and on in hummingbird fashion, and my heartbeat felt like it was being broadcast through a megaphone with a direct line to my ears. On Wednesday morning, the chemo fog rolled in. This was a feeling that I was enveloped in chemicals, and concentrating became a chore. Reading was out of the question. All I could do was stay in bed and stare at the TV. Whether it was on or off made no difference. Luckily this was lessened by the next day, but replaced by more heart palpitations and a feeling of dizziness like I had been slammed over the head with a cement block. This was all accompanied by a ravenous appetite, and despite the fact that I heaped my plate high with food all day long I had lost another three pounds. I also suffered from extreme thirst. In a given hour, I often had to consume up to 10 bottles of water to stave off the lightheadedness from dehydration, and at night, I would dream of sand being packed into my mouth, waking up to find my tongue a dry lump, stuck to the roof of my mouth. I was sure I now had diabetes.

By the time I went in for my blood work on Monday morning, I was a mess. My blood pressure was 180/120 and I thought I was going to pass out. When I told the nurse what was going on, she went to fetch the doctor. They looked at each other in that knowing way, and he asked if I had been taking the valium he had prescribed to me for anxiety, *like a good girl*, he may as well have added.

"This is NOT from anxiety," I protested, though at the moment I was having a full-blown panic attack. "This is from something you are giving me."

In the end, he agreed to lower the steroid that goes in my pre-med drip, handed me a prescription for Ativan, and another for high blood pressure, like a pat on the back. I imagined that they all sat around the break room talking about me, like I used to do with my fellow teachers that shared the same students. That was when I knew that I needed to take matters into my own hands.

I made a list of all the medications I now found myself on, and researched them one by one. What I discovered was that the steroid indeed could be responsible for my extreme thirst, ravenous appetite, heart palpitations, and weight loss. Being more sensitive to drugs than most people, this made some sense. I also discovered that the Neulasta was more than likely the cause of the dizziness, which was listed as an allergic reaction. There were going to have to be some changes. Otherwise, I did not think I could continue.

The rest of the week, being my week off of chemo, passed quite smoothly. My sister arrived all the way from Hawaii to give Jeff a much needed break from me and the craziness that we now lived in. The remainder of my hair had clogged up the drains, and I played with the different head coverings I had bought online. My brother also sent me an auburn colored wig. Since I looked nothing like me when I put it on, my sister and I named her "Claire." So Claire and my sister, in between naps, spent the week shopping, going to the movies, and even to the beach. But Sunday came all too fast, and the depression of facing Monday settled over me. That night, I enjoyed my first glass of wine in over a month as I tried to imagine myself a normal person, and prepared mentally for combat.

"I'm sending you for an MRI," the doctor said the next morning, when I again told him about the dizziness. "It is possible that you have brain cancer."

"*You do not have brain cancer,*" my sister mouthed behind his back.

"I do not have brain cancer," I told the doctor.

I had educated myself enough at that point to know that what he was saying was not actually as crazy as it might have sounded to my sister's ears. Triple negative breast cancer, if it comes back, often attacks the lungs, bones, and/or the brain. However, I also knew that cancer did not have a time clock.

"Since my symptoms occur regularly, say every Thursday at 7 p.m. during treatment week, wouldn't it be more likely that it is from one of the drugs that I am taking?" I asked logically.

"Maybe," he answered, "but we need to rule it out."

"What about the Neulasta," I said, showing him the print-out of side effects that include extreme dizziness.

"That is rare," he informed me, but then told me that there was another option – I could go on a lower dose of white blood cell boost called Neupogen which would be administered the following week over three days, but I wouldn't be able to have my last round of Adriamycin and Cytoxan (A/C) for another three weeks instead of two.

HALLELUEJAH!

I couldn't believe that this was the first time I was hearing about an option, but I was so relieved that I got over those feelings of dismay quickly. I would have three whole weeks! One week of the Chemoland rollercoaster, and then two entire weeks to feel almost normal. That meant that I could enjoy Thanksgiving, which was two weeks away. My excitement made sitting in The Big Chair not quite so painful that day.

When my sister and I left the chemo room three hours later, the receptionist was on the phone making me an appointment for the MRI which I had forgotten all about.

"I am going to hold off on the MRI for now," I told her.

I am extremely claustrophobic, and there was no way I was going to torture myself unnecessarily. This week would be the telling time if the dizziness was truly from the Neulasta shot or not. She had no problem with that, and I skipped out of the office and into what was left of the day.

The week that followed was a huge improvement. However, despite the lowered dose of steroids – from 20 milligrams to 10 – I still could not sleep that first night. This was partly because I was afraid that I would never wake up. When I did sleep, the nightmares were horrific. On Wednesday morning, the chemo fog rolled in and rendered me useless.

"It is just visiting," my sister assured me when I told her how horrible I felt.

And it was a short visit this time of only four hours. Thursday and Friday came and went, and I never got dizzy or had heart palpitations. My sister cooked for me all week, determined to get my white blood cell count up naturally, through food. This diet consisted of cheese and mushroom omelets with a side of strawberries in the morning, tuna sandwiches on whole grain bread for lunch, and fresh wild-caught fish with a side of sautéed baby spinach, and quinoa for dinner. By Sunday, I felt pretty normal.

"Keep doing what you are doing," the nurse said Monday morning when I had my blood work done. I was not going to need even the low dose white blood boost that week.

Sadly, after two short weeks, my sister went back to her life the next day, but I was looking forward to two whole weeks of normalcy. However, a few nights later I woke up with a fever and a toothache. When I saw the dentist the next day, he gave me some antibiotics, but said it would be best to have the tooth pulled. Despite the antibiotics, my fever continued to rise, and was at 101.6 by the time I saw the doctor a few days later.

He took a lot of blood, "to rule out sepsis (a blood infection), which would be disastrous," he said.

I wouldn't get those results for a few days, but he was able to tell me that my white blood cell count had dropped to 1.2%. The ideal number is 7.3%. Needless to say, I was given the low dose of white blood cell boost (Neupogen), and I would need to come back the following two days for more. If my count was high enough by the third day, I would have my tooth pulled. In the meantime, the doctor told me that if I got the chills or shakes, I should go directly to the ER. Just one more thing to add to my growing list of worries. The nightmares intensified.

I tolerated the Neupogen pretty well. I did have some bone pain, and felt slightly off balance for a couple of days, but nothing compared to how I had felt after Neulasta. Three days later, my tooth was pulled, and my fever immediately disappeared. I was frustrated that I had lost an entire week, but happy that the next day I was able to cook and enjoy our family Thanksgiving feast. I even had a glass of wine – I had a lot to be thankful for.

The next and final round of A/C went smoothly, but was accompanied by an entirely new set of side effects. I now found myself going through chemo-induced menopause, just as my friend Kim had promised. The hot flashes lasted all day long, but were bearable until nighttime, and I did not sleep much during those weeks. The heat was not like a fever; it was deep inside. And when the burning would stop, my body temperature would drop. The lowest I recorded was 96.4. The chemo nurse insisted that my thermometer was off when I discussed this with her, but after buying a new highly rated device, and taking my temperature using several different methods, the reading was the same. In fact, I became obsessed with taking my temperature. Between the burning hot flashes, and the feel of my ice cold flesh, I took an extensive log. I was also tired and weak, and spent a lot of time resting, but Christmas season was upon me, and I forced myself out of bed everyday to join the throng of shoppers. I was excited because my brother would be arriving in time for the holidays, and the next chemo treatment.

During those two weeks that I had off of chemo, I also began to research the new drug, Taxol, which I would be on for 12 consecutive weeks starting two days before Christmas. My oncologist had told me that most women tolerate Taxol much better than the

Adriamycin and Cytoxan combo that I was now done with. However, when I looked at the side effects of Taxol, I became alarmed. The biggest threat was an allergic reaction, which could lead to death. That was followed by neuropathy, which is nerve damage affecting the hands and feet, and also losing finger and toenails. Just when I had finally gotten down the whole A/C – steroid - white blood cell boost formula so that it was tolerable, it was now time to move on and face the next unknown, and I was terrified.

Chapter 5
Taxol, Taxane, Abraxane, It's All the Same

"There is a difference between giving up, and knowing when you have had enough."
— Robert Tew

My brother arrived the week before Christmas, and though I was still weak and tired, I felt pretty normal. We were able to enjoy shopping, eating out, and some days at the beach. I tried not to think about the week to come, which arrived way too soon. The fear of the unknown was all consuming, and I was depressed that I would more than likely have to spend Christmas in bed.

Despite my urge to flee, we arrived at the chemo room bright and early Monday morning. My chemo cocktail had changed drastically. The pre-meds now consisted of the low dose of steroid, and Benadryl. I explained to the nurse that I am extremely drug sensitive and perhaps 50 milligrams was going to be too much for me. However, after she reiterated what I already knew about Taxol and allergic reactions, we decided to go with the full dose. Benadryl was after all just an over-the-counter allergy remedy. What was there to be afraid of? However, for me this was a bad choice for the moment, but may have saved my life. As soon as the Benadryl hit my veins, I knew it was not going to be pretty, and I called out for the nurse.

"I think I am going to be sick," I told her, and she rushed off for a container.

I never threw up, but my body started to shake uncontrollably. It started with my legs, which were jerking about like someone had turned on a switch, and I couldn't find the off button. Then my stomach started to tremble, and the shaking continued up to my shoulders, and through my teeth which were chattering away. All through this, I struggled to stay awake as the Benadryl took over completely. I felt like a drowning Eveready battery.

Soon, I was surrounded by every chemo nurse on duty. One held my left hand, and my brother took the other. Another was massaging my right leg, and another my left. The last one was behind me, rubbing my shoulders, and leading me through breathing exercises. Anyone that glanced over might have thought that my moans were out of ecstasy. Waves of nausea rushed over me, tears sprang to my eyes, and I thought it would never end. But like all things, it did subside about 30 minutes later. The chemo nurses then retreated, leaving me alone with my jumbled thoughts, and my poor brother, who had come out from Seattle to spend Christmas with me and my family and endure this one chemo experience, which turned out to be the worst of them all.

"Are you ready to start the Taxol?" the main chemo nurse said to me after she had had a significant break.

"Ready as I will ever be," I answered in slurred speech, still reeling from the Benadryl.

And the dreaded chemo came down the line. This time the sensations started from the top down. At first, my nose felt tingly, and then my lips went numb. Soon after, it felt like an elephant was resting upon my chest. I was just about to call out for the nurse when this passed, and the only residue left was the usual heaviness in my legs. After six long hours, we were free to go. The nurse handed me a list of natural supplements to help with neuropathy if I were to get it, and recommended tea tree oil in case I had trouble with my finger or toenails which can be applied to the nails to harden them. She also suggested a mouth wash called Biotene in case I developed mouth sores. I decided to start using everything right away as a preventative measure, and we set off for the vitamin shop. Here is the list:

Vitamin B-Complex (I chose the one with biotin – which promotes hair growth)
Alpha Lipoic Acid
L-Carnatine
Glutamine
I also added CoQ10 which is for the heart

The glutamine came in a powder, so I also picked up a supply of vanilla whey protein, and began making fresh fruit smoothies every day. This is my favorite recipe:

1/2 cup coconut water
1/2 cup crushed ice
1 scoop vanilla whey protein
1 scoop glutamine
1 tablespoon coconut oil
6 fresh strawberries
1/2 banana
Put all ingredients in a blender, and mix till smooth

The week that followed was not so bad. I stayed in bed the remainder of that first day, and the next, which probably had more to do with a Benadryl hangover than the actual chemo. By Christmas morning, I was able to put on a real smile and enjoy time with my family. The next day, I was spent, and the constipation of the A/C days was replaced by diarrhea. The one nice thing about Taxol is that the white cell boost is typically not necessary, so I could put that old fear to rest. By the next Monday, my brother had left, and Jeff was back as my chemo buddy.

"I heard that the Benadryl made you a bit antsy," said the doctor that morning.

"Antsy?" I said. "I don't think that's exactly how I would describe it…"

"Well, we can lower your dosage to 12.5 instead of 50," he said.

Then I went on to tell him about the unusual sensations I had had during the infusion.

"That sounds like an allergic reaction," he informed me.

And therefore, a huge dilemma. If I took a lower dose of Benadryl, it may not be enough to counteract the allergy, which could possibly put my life at risk, and I was not willing to go through the high dose "antsy" experience on a weekly basis.

"You could opt out of chemo," he said, and my insides warmed with true happiness.

"Or we could try to get you approved for Abraxane," he offered.

The classification for this type of chemo is Taxane. There are three of them under the umbrella: Taxol, Taxotere, and Abraxane. Abraxane is said to be by far the kindest chemo of the three. It still comes along with the possibility of neuropathy, but it is typically so well tolerated that it can be given in higher doses, and does not pose the threat of allergic reactions like the other two, and therefore Benadryl is out of the equation. The problem is that it is very expensive and usually reserved for stage IV patients. Getting insurance approval seemed highly unlikely. In the end, we decided that he would try, and I would come back in two weeks to learn my fate.

Those two weeks were bittersweet. I felt great, and was able to go to the gym, and the best news of all was that my hair had started to grow. But I suffered internally. On the one hand, I was elated at the prospect of no more chemo, but how could I know if the A/C had been enough? There was no way to tell. I resigned myself to the fact that chemo was over for good, and I would just have to believe that it had done the job. Those 14 days flew by, but were soon replaced with more appointments.

"Your Abraxane has been approved!" the doctor told me, and my heart sank.

I knew this was supposed to be good news, but over the last two weeks, I had convinced myself that even if the Abraxane had been miraculously approved, I would decline. I was feeling too great to go back now.

"Oh," I stammered, stalling for time. "I can't do it today. I'm not prepared," I told him, meaning that I had to think about it, and besides, I hadn't brought any of my supplies, and more importantly, no one was there to hold my hand.

"Well, next week for sure," he declared, and I was set free to mull things over.

Over the next few days, I spent hours on the internet researching Taxanes and triple negative breast cancer. I was looking for statistics that would nullify my need to have one, and make me feel better about my decision to back out. However, the research was not cooperating with me. From everything I read, it was bitterly clear that Abraxane would absolutely improve my chances of ultimate survival.

When the information had a chance to settle in, it was really a no-brainer. How could I say no to this opportunity and be able to face myself in the mirror? What would I tell my daughter if I refused, and the cancer came back? Then I thought of all the women, huddled under their blankets, asleep in the chemo room getting their Taxol who would jump at this offer. Abraxane was a gift, and of course I would do it.

So Monday morning, I once again found myself back in The Big Chair with Jeff there to hold my hand, and tote my supplies. When I found out that my pre-meds would still consist of steroids, I convinced the chemo nurse to lower the dose even further to five milligrams. Since I had never had any nausea, she agreed. Abraxane takes time to mix properly, and waiting for it was a lot longer than the infusion itself. When it finally arrived, it looked a lot more like milk than a cocktail.

Once it started to drip, I took out a bag of frozen peas. I had been reading about Penguin Caps, which are given out at some chemo facilities. The idea is that if you freeze your hair follicles, the chemo can't do any harm, and I was determined not to lose the $1/6^{th}$ of an inch of hair that I currently had on my head. I placed the frozen pea pack in a ski cap, and wore it during the 30 minute infusion. I also held frozen water bottles in my hands in the hopes of preventing neuropathy. I got some funny looks from the nurse, but she didn't say a word. I'm sure they have seen all sorts of crazy contraptions. Or maybe not.

The criteria for what constituted a "good day" were completely altered from what they had been before I entered Chemoland. In my real life, a good day meant that I met friends for coffee in the morning, put in a solid three to four hours of writing, picked up my daughter from school, took the dogs for a walk, went to the gym, cooked dinner, and spent the evening with my family. In Chemoland, a "good day" meant that I was able to pick my daughter up from school, walk the dogs, and make dinner.

For the first few weeks on Abraxane, the side effects were minimal, and I was actually able to enjoy some great days. I had a stuffy nose, and then a runny nose. I was tired more often than not, and the hot flashes continued, but this I could do. During this time, I was able to go to the gym and do a reduced workout, take a beginning photography class, and I even managed to publish my first novel, which was a children's animal adventure story, and being immersed in that world every day was a very welcome distraction. The biggest issue I had was that my finish line to getting out of Chemoland kept getting pushed back. The Abraxane schedule differed from the Taxol. Instead of 12 consecutive weeks, I would get chemo three weeks in a row, and then have one week off. But if that was all I had to complain about, life was good.

Until the midway point that is. It all started with pain on the tops of my feet on a Wednesday morning. The following week, the pain travelled up my legs and lasted through Thursday. The week after, I was just in pain. It became difficult to walk, and then I began having headaches. After that, I started feeling seasick all of the time. The ground would often come up to meet me and I would trip over it, so I mostly stayed in bed. I also noticed that the little hair I had started to thin out significantly. I had abandoned the pea pack during treatment at about the halfway point. Who knows if it would have fallen out anyway. Toward the end of treatment, I had about one hair for every 1000 follicles, and the ones that remained were about one inch long. I looked like a pathetic version of a grown kewpie doll. The biggest consolation was that I was counting down the weeks to crossing that finish line, and soon I only had two to go.

There were three major events that I saw to be common amongst cancer patients going through chemo that I was determined to avoid. One was a blood transfusion which treats low red blood cell production, and thankfully, that was never an issue for me. The second was an MRI, and I had skirted around that one. The third was a trip to the ER.

On that second to last chemo day, everything seemed to be going well. Jeff and I arrived early as usual, and ironically, for the first time ever, my blood pressure was within the normal range. The chemo nurse even commented on how calm I had become compared to the early days. But the last thing I felt that day was calm. I knew that something was wrong, but there was nothing specific to report. I just felt uncomfortable in my own skin, and like I shouldn't be there. The urge to yank out the IV was strong, but I had no words to justify it. I tried to distract myself by reading, but I couldn't focus on the words. I tried to play a game, but I couldn't concentrate. I got up and went to the bathroom several times because I was having a hard time sitting still. When the infusion was finally over, I couldn't get out of there fast enough.

By the time we got home, the "off" feeling had subsided and I went to bed, seasick and groggy as usual. A couple of hours later, a dull ache started on the left side of my chest. Then my heart began doing calculated flip flops. This was much different from the fluttering that I had become used to in the A/C days. There was a definite pattern to it. It only lasted a few minutes, and because of my overall state of fogginess, I didn't think much of it. While living in Chemoland, I had become accustomed to bizarre physical reactions.

My head felt a little clearer by the next morning, though, and I decided to call the chemo nurse. She advised me to see my regular doctor ASAP. This alarmed me because previously my complaints had been brushed aside. My regular doctor, however, was on vacation, and I couldn't get an appointment for two weeks. The chemo nurse called back a couple of hours later to make sure I was going to be seen, and this distressed me further. When I told her the predicament, she insisted that I go to the dreaded emergency room.

Seven tubes of blood, an EKG, a chest x-ray, a CT scan, and six hours later, the attending ER physician diagnosed me with having had a chemo induced heart arrhythmia.

"I've seen it many times," he informed me, and strongly warned me against having any more chemo. He then wrote a note to my oncologist with this recommendation.

I only had one more to go, and I didn't want to be a quitter when I was so close, but I knew in my heart that he was right. I was certain that my body could not, and should not take any more. I then did the math, and it turned out that because Abraxane is given at a much higher dose than Taxol, I had actually already had more chemo than I would have had if I had remained on the Taxol for 12 weeks. It had been exactly six months from the first chemo infusion of A/C, and I was finally done.

Chapter 6
Tantrums

"Endurance is not just the ability to bear a hard thing, but to turn it into glory."
—William Barclay

Going through cancer treatment not only takes its toll physically, but also mentally and emotionally. One of the biggest hurdles for anyone, especially women going through chemo is the bald factor. The one and only time during all of this craziness that I cried was early on, before I lost my hair, and had taken a trip to the wig store. As soon as the kind lady asked how she could help me, much to my own surprise, I burst into tears and left.

Many women I knew in the chemo room never covered their heads at all. In a way, I envied them, but I was much too vain, or perhaps it was that I lacked the confidence. I had the one wig that my brother had sent, and I wore it on special occasions, and on some days to the supermarket just for the fun of it. But mostly I did not wear it because it was hot and itchy, and more importantly made me feel "not me". I had ordered bandanas from Amazon, and in the beginning I wore those until they became boring. Then I ordered five beanies from curediva.com. But in the end, I only wore two of those regularly because they were silky, soft, and felt good on my head.

The problem for me was that one of them was pink paisley, and the other was red. This became a fashion nightmare, and a big source of my tantrums. I would stand in my closet, and throw my shirts on the ground one by one in frustration until my ankles were swimming me in a sea of colors, and I knew that only I would be the one to bring order to the chaos. The only shirts that would go with pink or red were the white ones, and I was sick of wearing white. This was even worse on chemo days because it is necessary to wear a V-neck, so that the nurse could access my port. I thought that this might be a good excuse to go shopping, but trying to match that particular shade of pink and red was impossible, and I refused to invest more money in those head coverings because I was not going to need them soon. As time went on, I quit caring. I could often be seen with a pink head, and an orange top, looking like a badly dyed Easter egg, or with a bright red beanie and green shirt, like a misplaced Christmas elf.

Another pet peeve I had was when people would tell me how "good" I looked. This well-meaning comment somehow infuriated me. I was 10 pounds underweight, making me look sickly and pale. My face had sunken in, and I had dark circles under my eyes. And I was bald. There was nothing "good" about the way I looked. It also insinuated to me, however irrationally, that the speaker thought that I must be having an easy time in Chemoland. So I would invariably hit the poor do-gooder with one of my latest horror stories: my bad reaction to the Benadryl, the allergic reaction to Taxol, or my trip to the ER. Would I really have preferred for someone to say to me, "Hey, Tamzen! You look like crap."? Maybe.

It also bothered me when friends would tell me how "brave" I was. There was absolutely nothing brave about me. I lived in total fear. Fear of what the chemo was doing to me, fear of what was next, fear that my hair would never come back, and fear of dying. On any given day, not 10 minutes would go by that I did not think about cancer and death. I was the epitome of a chicken. The worst for me, though, was meeting new people because the person they were seeing for the first time was not me.

"You are still you," Jeff would say, but I wasn't convinced.

I was the woman with long golden hair, and a healthy body weight. I was the woman that went to the gym four times a week, enjoyed hiking and kayaking, cooking, and family road trips. I did not recognize this person that I had become. Oftentimes I would have to resist the urge to pull up "before" pictures on my phone, to prove to them that this was not me. But I didn't want to be like those new mothers that post a zillion pictures of their newborn every day on social media. After all, no one really cared what I looked like before, except me. This identity crisis lasted long after I had thrown out all of the head coverings and sported my very own full head of very short, thick blond hair.

"I am sick of being tired, tired of being sick, and over being bald," I complained to my daughter one day.

"Stop whining," was her response.

After I resisted the urge to smack her, I thought about it from her perspective. I needed to remind myself that this was almost as hard on my family as it was on me. Jeff had accompanied me to all of my visits to The Big Chair, with the exception of the two that I had had my siblings with me. He also took at least one other day off of work during the week when I knew I would need help. His job was suffering, and so was his mental health, along with mine.

My daughter was basically without a mother for that entire year. I did not attend most of her school events, and she became responsible for cooking her own dinner, and making sure the dogs got walked regularly. I had no idea where she went after school, and on weekends, or how she got there. She never complained about these things, so I knew that I had no right to either. It was time to put on my happy face.

The following Monday, I met a woman in the elevator while I was on my way up to the chemo room. She had gone through treatment a year earlier, and now led the local program "Look Good, Feel Better," which is sponsored by the American Cancer Society. She handed me a brochure, and I signed up the next day. It was the best thing I did for myself so far.

There were seven other women there for the class that day. And they all were bald! It felt for me like coming home. For an hour we practiced putting on makeup, trying on wigs, telling stories, and laughing. Although we began as complete strangers, by the end we felt just like sisters. When our session was up, we were each given a bountiful package of top-of-the-line cosmetics, and a wig of our choice. Mine was short, blonde, and sassy, and I named her Samantha.

After that, I started to venture out even more. I found that the cancer center held monthly yoga classes, and I attended when I could. The women there were in different stages of treatment - some with no hair, some with stubbles like mine, and others with locks down to their shoulders. Friends and family were a great support, but Chemoland became much more bearable when there were people in my life that could relate on a base level to exactly what I was going through. I continued with this class long after I was finished with treatment for both the camaraderie, and because it was a great class.

Chapter 7
The Great Radiation Debate

"Man is a creature that can get used to anything, and I think that is the best definition of him."
— Fyodor Dostoyevsky

Before I had the lumpectomy, my surgeon had referred me to a Radiation Oncologist to discuss the option of internal versus external radiation. If I opted for the internal route, called balloon-catheter internal radiation, a balloon would need to be placed at the surgery site during the lumpectomy. This type of radiation takes place over only one week, with two treatments per day. In the end, I decided to go with the traditional external radiation because there was not enough research on the long term effectiveness of this relatively new internal variation.

During the course of that visit, the Radiation Oncologist informed me that smokers, and even former smokers, are twice as likely as non-smokers to develop lung cancer years after receiving radiation for breast cancer. This information nagged at me throughout my time in Chemoland, and I constantly debated not going through with this phase of treatment. I also couldn't really understand from a logical standpoint the necessity of it. If chemo had chased down any stray cancer cells throughout my entire body, then why do radiation? Did they think it hadn't worked? These were questions that I brought to the table when I met with my second

Radiation Oncologist a few days after chemo was finished.

At our initial meeting, she assured me that radiation was indeed the best option for me, but I couldn't help thinking that of course she would say that. When I brought up my concern of lung cancer, she informed me that the chances of developing a secondary tumor were minuscule, and that while it is true that smokers are twice as likely to have this happen, it is still less than a fraction of a percent likely – still at minutia levels. She also explained to me that while chemo does indeed attack cancer cells throughout the body, there is a much greater chance of having a stray cell at the surgery site, and therefore, radiation was like a double insurance plan for not having a recurrence. That made sense to me, so I signed on that day.

I had four weeks between the last chemo infusion and the official start of radiation, and my body was more than ready for a break. However, during that time, and much to my distress, the chemo side effects got worse; something that no one had told me was a possibility. This lack of information caused me a lot of needless mental anguish. I was constantly dizzy, had intense headaches, earaches, and developed ringing and a muffling in my right ear. Of course, I was convinced that I had brain cancer after all. Instead, I had nerve damage in my inner ear, which luckily turned out to be temporary. The worst of it lasted about three weeks.

Then my fingers and toes went numb, then stiff, and became painful. This often kept me up at night, but I discovered that if I took an Aleve right before bed, I could make it through the night. Once I moved around in the morning, it mostly went away. However, after a few weeks, the stiffness traveled to my elbows, shoulders and knees. I was now convinced that I had bone cancer. Instead, I had developed chemo induced neuropathy and a case of osteoarthritis. This peaked two months later and then slowly began to subside.

The morning that I was to begin radiation, I woke up knowing that something was different. The heavy fog that had engulfed me for many months had lightened - just a little, but enough to make me elated. I was still lethargic, and my joints continued to bother me, but

I could immediately tell the difference. It was the hope that I had been waiting for; that eventually, I would be normal. I immediately got on the computer and booked a celebration trip to Key Largo for the end of treatment which would also be my daughter's 16th birthday. Then I drove to the cancer center with a new outlook.

The radiation office, though it was in the same building as the chemo room, had a much different feel. It was much larger and with fewer patients, there were coffee and cookies neatly arranged on the granite counter, and the furnishings were modern and comfortable. Compared to the hectic nature of the chemo room, it was almost soothing.

"I will be your therapist," said the young woman who greeted me in the waiting room that morning. Though that is what these technicians call themselves, the patients commonly referred to them as "The Zappers."

My therapist then escorted me into the dressing room which was complete with robes, lockers for my clothing, a key that I could wear around my wrist, and a sitting room with a television. I was hopeful that she would next lead me into the massage room, but instead, there was a huge machine, and I was told to lie down and hold my arms way above my head. For the next 45 minutes, my therapist and her assistants took pictures of my chest, drew ink spots that would eventually become permanent tattoos, and instructed me to stay still. That was the hardest part. When I left an hour later, I was told that starting the following Monday I would get radiation every day at 11 a.m. for six weeks. I was cautioned against putting anything on the right side of my body such as powder, perfume, lotion, or deodorant prior to treatment. I was also told to altogether stay away from deodorant that contained aluminum. I found a great substitute for my usual Secret, called Crystal Essence, which I still use.

During the first session, I again had to hold my arms over my head for another 45 minutes while my therapist made sure that all of the tattoos lined up perfectly with the machines. After that, each treatment was only 90 seconds. Top 40 music pumped through the speakers as the machine swept over me. It would start at the right side of my breast where the lumpectomy scar resided, pause for 30 seconds, then move directly on top of me for another 30 seconds, and then sweep to the left for the final 30 seconds. I would stare at the ceiling which had a painting of a white sand beach, and count backwards slowly from 90. Then I would be released back into the dressing room to change, and go on with my day.

After six months of treatment, and countless medical professionals looking at my breasts, modesty had gone out the window a long time ago. I often had to be reminded to close my robe for the few steps back to the dressing room because the men's quarters were just to the right.

Radiation was like going on vacation in Iowa after having been a POW in the Middle East. I envied the women in the waiting room with full heads of hair that were also there for treatment, and obviously never had to take the journey through the Chemoland nightmare. But then again, perhaps Iowa was more distasteful to them than it was for me.

After only a few days into the first week, my chest on the left side where my port was placed began to ache, and I worried that I had a blood clot. I brought this up to the radiation oncologist. She looked at it and declared there was nothing wrong. I then told my therapist, who said it was probably a result of holding my arms over my head for an extended period, and to have it checked at the oncologist's office.

I was scheduled for a port flush the following week, so decided to wait until then. This was something that had to be done once a month since my port was no longer being used. Over the week, the pain began to increase, especially when I exercised. I had started taking a Pilates class, and was again walking my dogs everyday. The chemo nurse affirmed that there was nothing wrong with my port which she was able to flush easily.

The pain intensified, and was now throbbing. Just putting on my seatbelt was difficult, and I would have to place the shoulder strap under my arm where it wouldn't rub against my port. The ache now kept me up at night, and I wanted that thing out.

"It's up to your oncologist," my radiation oncologist told me, so I made an appointment with him.

"It's up to your radiation oncologist," he told me after inspecting my port and also telling me there was nothing wrong.

My thinking was that if a foreign object in my body hurt, it must come out, so I went straight to the source. The surgeon asked me how long it had been hurting, and when I told him it had been almost a month, he asked why I still had it in.

"Because no one wants to be responsible for making the call to take it out," I answered.

"Nonsense! I'll take it out tomorrow," he declared.

And so he did. Though this procedure still required fasting the night before and a trip to the surgery center, taking it out was even easier than putting it in. I opted to be awake for the surgery, and although I was sedated, I was aware of everything going on. The whole operation took about 20 minutes, and since I wasn't put under, the recovery was very quick. I now had a scar across my right chest, too, but the pain from the port was immediately gone forever.

At about the half way point in my radiation therapy, while the chemo fog continued to roll out of my life, radiation fatigue started to move in. Despite this, I was able to continue my Pilates class twice a week, and take a brisk walk every day. I found that a 45 minute nap in the afternoon easily took care of it. Then the promised radiation burn began to appear. At first, my entire breast turned pink. Then underneath it, the skin began to crack and peel. I was given a heavy duty thick cream to apply at night called Aquaphor, and during the day I soothed it with the aloe plant that grew in my back yard. This was a winning combination. I also noticed that when I exercised, my arms and legs would feel like they were being pricked by a million tiny pins. I was told that this is normal.

The worst part about radiation was not the treatment itself. It seemed that my body had a natural aversion to the sight of the cancer center, and every time I drove up, my blood pressure would rise. Even when I felt like I was calm, the readings were off the charts, and I began to worry. The first time they took it, the reading was 150/105. The nurse told me to retake it later in the day, which I did. I was troubled about the high numbers, and even on my own, it was 150/100. I had been taking it regularly since the start of chemo, and at the beginning it was 115/70. Halfway through chemo it was 120/80. Now the best I got was 115/84. It seemed that chemo had permanently raised my blood pressure.

A week later, the nurse took it again, and it registered 170/114. At that time, she made a note in my chart that said, "White Coat Hypertension". The official diagnosis. Then she quit taking it altogether. I did, however, and it never got lower than 115/84.

The best part about radiation was that my hair had really started to come in. When it had been exactly two months since my last chemo infusion, and about a month into radiation, I gathered up all of my bandanas, head scarves, beanies and wigs. I put them in a box which I stored in the garage, only to possibly pull out on Halloween. Though the downy layer that had grown on my head was still sparse, and what my daughter referred to as "penguin feathers," I didn't care anymore. It was June in Florida, and the air was already hot and heavy. It was so liberating to walk out into the world natural. Once I made the decision, it felt like overnight that I developed a thick head of blond curls. I was ecstatic, though I still had somewhat of an identity crisis. Secretly, I thought my short hair was kind of cute, just not on me. It would have looked really good on someone else, like someone who chose to have short hair.

On the last day of treatment, I was given a crisp certificate of completion. I felt kind of cheated that I didn't get one at the end of chemo, but since I opted out of the last infusion, I never officially completed it. In the end, I didn't hang this one up on my wall, proud of my accomplishment. It now lives in the bottom drawer of my desk in a bright pink folder that I had been given on the day of my diagnosis labeled "All Things Cancer".

Chapter 8
The "New" Normal

"Fear never prevents anyone from dying; only from living."
— Unknown

The end of cancer treatment was anticlimactic for me. It was like how I imagined it would be to get out of prison after a very long time. The doors open, and you walk out into the big wide world, not knowing where to go or how to get there, and feeling a bit lost. I was so used to seeing doctors every day, and being poked, squeezed, and prodded, that now, I didn't know what to do with myself. Everything had just stopped.

I still had to see my team of medical professionals every three months, but I was essentially free – out on my own. This should have made me euphoric, but I had become afraid of my own body which pretty much made me still a prisoner.

"When will I be normal?" I would ask anyone that might have a clue.

The answers varied greatly.

"In about six months," I was told.

"Within a year," was another answer.

"You will find your "new" normal," I heard from many, and this was the answer that I hated the most.

I didn't even want to know what a "new" normal meant. I wanted my "old" normal. I wanted to be myself, and I wanted it

NOW. However, as time went on, I began to understand this foreign concept more and more, and I was determined to make my "new" normal better than the old one. This started with taking an inventory of my battle wounds, including, physical, mental and emotional scars, and then working on them one by one until they were solved to the greatest extent, and then learning to live with what remained.

Physically, I still had stiff joints, and I found that the more I exercised, the less they bothered me. I also suffered from chemo induced menopausal symptoms, especially vaginal dryness which boiled down to very painful intercourse, and none of my doctors wanted to prescribe anything for me even though my tumor had not been estrogen positive. Our sex life had already taken a big hit from the moment of diagnosis. We had made love only once during treatment – right before I lost my hair. After that, aside from feeling like crap most of the time, being bald really put a damper on the sexy factor. Once treatment was finished, because it had been so long, love making became almost awkward. We fumbled like self-conscious teenagers which might have been fun even without the benefit of raging hormones, but intimacy now came with a burning reward. We tried all of the usual suspects like Astroglide and KY, but not even they could provide an oasis in my barren desert.

I began researching natural supplements, and found an over-the-counter remedy called Menoquil. It had great reviews, and no side effects. I also still suffered from fatigue, which three months after chemo had ended, seemed to be getting worse. The question was if it was still a reaction from a chemo hangover, or was it related to menopause. Either way, it needed to be solved because it was becoming debilitating. I had become a zombie, and no amount of sleep revived me.

Menoquil seemed like the best solution. However, in the medical world, there is some controversy over one of the ingredients – soy isoflavones which are plant substances chemically similar to the female hormone estrogen. When I asked my team of medical professionals for advice, I got three different answers. One said it was fine. Another strongly recommended that I do not take it until there is further research, and the third did not express an opinion either way. I then read dozens of research studies on soy isoflavones, and they were inconsistent. Some warn against taking it because it acts like estrogen, and therefore may increase the likelihood of estrogen positive breast cancer though this has not been proven. Others actually concluded that it might help prevent breast cancer, and other studies suggest that it has no effect one way or the other. I decided to go ahead and take it, but only a half dose. Ten days later, I felt a huge improvement in my energy level.

As it had been throughout my time in Chemoland, the biggest issue for me was my mental state. Some lucky people are able to skip through anything life gives them seemingly undaunted, but for most people who have faced a deadly disease, their psyche is altered. I was one of the unlucky ones and maybe more of an extremist. I thought about death every 10 minutes of every waking hour for over a year

The truth is that I was afraid to adjust my thoughts. I believed that if I didn't appreciate the gravity of the situation enough, I would be in denial. My new superstitious self thought that if I continued to live care free, I would jinx myself, and the cancer would return. I believed that I should suffer because many women lose their lives to breast cancer every day, and I shouldn't feel like I had gotten away with anything. I knew it could happen to anyone, and could come back anytime, and I needed to be ready. As ridiculous as that sounds to me now, I lived with this way of thinking day in and day out for over a year. I also knew that when I ended treatment, it was time to change my thought pattern, but I didn't know how. The answer came gradually.

From the beginning of this journey, I saw over and over how powerful the mind is and how that affects the body. Until now, this had all been through negative encounters. It was time to get back my optimistic nature and use this power for the affirmative. If stressful thoughts could lead to high blood pressure, and excessive worry was followed by severe panic attacks that took over physically, then it seemed logical to me that positive thinking could only lead to good outcomes. I wasn't naïve enough to necessarily think that happy fuzzy thoughts could stop cancer from growing, but I did know that they would make living in my skin a much better place to be.

I started by taking a meditation class that was offered every week for free at the local yoga studio. I was taught several breathing techniques which focused energy on any problematic tension. It was obvious that my body had become a high voltage danger zone of stress; it buzzed, and hummed, and twitched and jerked uncontrollably, and at first, sitting still in a meditative state was disturbing. I felt sorry for the others in the class who were trying to relax. To supplement this, I took a hot bath every night before bed to help me sleep through the night. After a few weeks, the stress that I had been carrying for over a year began to slowly dissipate.

Through this class, while being taught the practice of meditation, I also discovered how to control my caustic thoughts. When I detected a negative thought bubble forming in my head, I would mentally shoo it out into the universe before it would have a chance to become identifiable words. Once out in thin air, it would pop and disintegrate without ever solidifying. In the beginning, this was very time consuming as the destructive clouds poured into my brain. By letting these negative thoughts roam around in my head unchecked for so long, they had been multiplying. Now they were effectively being destroyed.

I also practiced a visualization technique every day. This involved lying down, and relaxing each part of my body one by one. Then I would imagine what I would describe as fairy dust sweeping through my body to clean out any negative energy, or pollution. The purple sparkles would enter through the top of my head and whisk around my brain. Then they would travel through my arms, my torso, and down through my legs and feet, cleansing my entire system.

Making lifestyle changes was also a big part of getting to my new and improved normal. Obviously, cigarettes would need to be out of my life forever. I had quit five times during treatment, which also meant I had started five times. It was time to admit that I could not do it alone, so I asked for a prescription for Chantix. I also purchased an electronic cigarette, and loads of nicotine gum. It was time to win this battle once and for all.

I also found that exercise is beneficial in so many ways. For one, it actually increased my waning energy level. Furthermore, the National Cancer institute reports that "there is strong evidence that physical activity is associated with reduced risk of cancers of the colon and breast." The Centers for Disease Control and Prevention (CDC) recommend that adults "engage in moderate-intensity physical activity for at least 30 minutes on five or more days of the week," or "engage in vigorous-intensity physical activity for at least 20 minutes on three or more days of the week." To this tune, I returned to the gym to do a cardio workout three days a week, and I continued to take Pilates and yoga, and to practice meditation.

Another big lifestyle change that is important for fighting cancer is diet. Today, 1 in 8 women will develop breast cancer in their lifetime. 50 years ago, this statistic was 1 in 11. It is also a fact that the incidence of breast cancer is highest in more developed countries and lowest in less developed countries. While there is no firm data as to why this is, it makes sense to me that it is due to environmental changes. At this point in my life, I do not have a lot of control over the environment, but I can dictate what I put into my body.

I had never paid much attention to the food that I ate before, but now I read all of the labels, and made a point to research diet and cancer. Little by little, all of the food in my refrigerator and in my cupboards turned to organic. I wanted to know that everything I consumed was edible. I didn't need chemicals on my fruits and vegetables. I exchanged margarine for butter. When I purchased fish, I made sure it was wild-caught as opposed to farmed. I checked that the chicken and eggs I put on my plate were raised free-range, grass-fed and contained no antibiotics. I limited my red meat intake. I cut out fast food, and I no longer had sugary drinks, except wine. I am not a saint.

Next it was time to concentrate on my emotions. One might argue that it is impossible to change one's feelings, but I entirely disagree. I firmly believe that our perception of an event dictates our mind-set. If going to the cancer center were always a negative experience, then of course driving up to it would be met with distaste which can manifest itself physically (perhaps high blood pressure), emotionally (maybe tears), and mentally (horrific thoughts). However, if I changed my perception, and embraced my treatment, wholly convinced that whatever I was going to physically experience was beneficial, such as believing that it was saving my life, then perhaps driving up to the cancer center would invoke feelings of gratefulness. It is also possible to consciously conjure up positive feelings. If I get in my car, and pretend that I am excited about going to see my oncologist, my body will react to the excitement physically, and thus become real.

I now was armed with all of these great new tools, and it was time to put them to the test. Three months after I finished radiation, I was scheduled for a chest x-ray, a mammogram, and a PET scan. Two days after I was to get my results, I would be flying to San Diego to meet my brother and my sister to celebrate her 50th birthday. All of which were terrifying events for me. My first reaction was to reschedule all of these tests until after the trip. If anything came up cancer, I didn't want to spoil my sister's party. However, I knew that this was my old way of thinking, and I had done a lot of work toward my "new" normal. I had to face myself and my fears. Jeff offered to come with me, but this I needed to do alone.

It had been exactly one year since the first PET scan, and everything was exactly the same, down to the technician, but the experience itself was vastly different. My biggest worry was that I would be worried. I again sat alone in a small room and was injected with radioactive dye. The hour passed quickly while I rested, and then I was led into the room with the big machine. Although the process was exactly the same, I was calm, and it seemed to go very quickly. I concentrated on the music that was playing in the background, and not the reason that I was there, or the possible results.

"So I guess I'll never see you again," the technician said when it was over, and those were the best possible words I could hear.

The chest x-ray was a breeze, and only the mammogram challenged my power of positive thinking.

"You are probably getting an ultrasound anyway," the nurse said after releasing my breast from the vice grip.

She left the room to have the images read, and that word "anyway" had plenty of time to take up residence in my brain. I began to sweat, and the walls crept closer. Over and over, I visualized her coming back into the room with a smile on her face and saying the words, "everything looks good!" I must have gone through this scenario 1,000,000 times because she was gone for what seemed like forever.

"Who was your surgeon?" she asked when she finally made a reappearance.

These weren't exactly the words I had been hoping for, but they were better than "we are sending you for an ultrasound."

She then frowned instead of smiled, and checked my scar.

"The doctor wanted me to make sure that you really had a lumpectomy," she explained.

As if I could ever make this crap up! Couldn't she see my short hair?

"I don't get it," I said, wondering if this was some kind of joke.

"The surgery site is so clean," she said. "Your surgeon didn't leave behind any markers, and there is no scar tissue."

I had to laugh. Of all the compliments I had received regarding what a great job he had done, this was over the top. He was going to love it.

A short week later, I drove to the cancer center for the results. "Let it Be," was playing on the radio which seemed appropriate, and I turned it up full blast, singing my way through the short ride. I was surprised when a couple of stray tears of raw emotion sprang to my eyes as I approached the parking lot.

I waited in the cramped lobby, and looked around. There were new and old faces, bald heads, and others with long hair. Some of the nurses I didn't recognize, but the frenzied atmosphere was the same. I had come a long way since I had been a regular here. I was soon called back to the doctor's office by a nurse that I had known from the beginning.

"You look great!" she said, and I believed her.

She took my blood for the routine tumor marker tests and left me alone to wait. After I had visualized the doctor walking in the room 1,000 times saying "everything looks good!" he arrived. But those were not his words.

"You look great!" he said, mimicking the nurse.

I appreciated his sentiment, but I wanted to get down to business.

"I am here for my results," I said, motioning to his computer monitor where I knew the truth lay.

He took my lead, and scrolled through the reports, pausing every now and then.

"You had a mammogram last week, and every thing was fine, right?" he asked, though the results were right before his eyes.

"Yes," I answered impatiently.

"And the chest x-ray looks good," he said.

The surgeon's office had called the day before, confirming both of these results already.

"And the PET scan?" I asked, trying to move him along to what I was really here for.

"There was some activity in your right breast..." he said, not looking up.

My right breast? The one and same that I had just gone through all this for?

My eyes shot daggers across the room, though they were not meant for him. I didn't realize before that I could add "anger" to my list of negative emotions.

"...though this is consistent with radiation therapy recently received," he continued reading. "Probably scar tissue forming," he concluded.

So the scar tissue had arrived after all.

Two days later, I boarded my flight to San Diego. This was another mental challenge for me. I had always been terrified of flying, and this was the first time since my daughter was born that I would be doing it solo – without a hand to squeeze. I sat back in my seat, and visualized a bright blue protective halo surrounding the plane. Then I conjured up what it would feel like to be a kid visiting Disneyland for the first time. Excitement! Yes. I was determined to feel excited about this flight. And I had a lot to be thrilled about. All of my tests came back clear, I was done with treatment, and I was going to spend a fun-filled week with my siblings. As we circled around the Dallas airport for 45 minutes, and the airplane shuddered and swerved in the heavy winds, I imagined that I was coasting down the slopes of the Matterhorn. Finally we landed, and the excitement was real. The next flight into San Diego was uneventful, and I had made it.

Three days into my vacation I would be put to the real test and fail miserably. My phone rang, and when I looked at the incoming phone number, saw it was the oncologist's office. I had forgotten to worry about the tumor marker tests. I began to sweat, and my hands began to shake. That phone number to me spelled D-E-A-T-H, so I let the call go to voice mail. I took a few moments to gather my courage, and then headed out to the beach by myself. I knew I had to listen to that message, but I didn't want to ruin our trip. It took all the inner strength I had to push that button and play back the call. It was the nurse calling to let me know that my Chantix prescription was ready. I was immediately relieved, but also disappointed in myself for my physical reaction. I was definitely a work in progress.

Chapter 9
Words of Wisdom

"By three methods we may learn wisdom: First, by reflection, which is noblest; Second, by imitation, which is easiest; and third by experience, which is the bitterest."
— Confucius

If I could go back and talk to my newly diagnosed self, I would have some advice. First, I would tell myself to **stay away from the internet**. Sure, the World Wide Web has its place, like when I wanted to understand my diagnosis more clearly, and when I needed to know the specific side effects of all of the medications I was taking. These things were real, and were happening, but I had done more than that. I had abused the search engines, and I was the only victim of this offense. At first it was about the numbers. I looked up every statistic I could find on cancer and survival rates to the point of obsession. The reality is that even before treatment, I had a much better chance of never seeing cancer again than I did of having a recurrence. Either it is going to happen or its not. I do not have control. My cup is more than half full, and that is what I needed to focus on.

I had also become insanely attuned to my body, and as a result of that, and with the help of the internet, killed myself off with a new self-diagnosed disease on a monthly basis. First it was heart failure. From the beginning of chemo, I had experienced palpitations and a racing heart, and was convinced that I was going to keel over any day, or worse, while I was sleeping. This kept me up many nights. After that, it was diabetes. My symptoms were extreme thirst and hunger, with progressive weight loss. This was all from the steroids. Next, I was certain that I had ovarian cancer; I had pain on the right side of my lower abdomen. It turned out to be gas. Then it was skin cancer. I had a large mole on my stomach that was changing shape. This was due to the chemotherapy – it was flaking off. I had it removed, and it came back benign. That was followed by breast cancer. I felt a lump in my left breast (the cancer had been in my right breast). I went for a mammogram, and it came back normal. After that, I gave myself brain cancer. I was getting bad headaches, earaches, vertigo, and then ringing in my ears; all a result of temporary nerve damage from chemo. Next, I convinced myself that I had a blood clot in my port, and that it was going to break off and go to my heart or lungs, and kill me. It was only a strained muscle attached to the port. After that, I had bone cancer – twice. I had pain in all of my joints, and my collar bone and legs ached. This turned out to be chemo related arthritis. Soon after, I developed two lumps on my right wrist. These were ganglion cysts from overuse– I had been sanding the floors. All of these deadly diseases were self diagnosed with the help of the internet, and none of them were real.

If I could go back, I would also tell myself to **ask for help**. By the time I started treatment, all of my friends that I had made in Florida were scattered across the country and beyond. This left only Jeff and my daughter as my support group. However, a slew of neighbors had stopped by to offer their support and phone numbers in case I needed anything. Even though Jeff was two hours away at work on most days, I never called, and I should have. On some days, I could have used someone to bring me a fresh sandwich. On other days, it would have been nice to have had some company. But I was too wrapped up in my own Hell to reach out. The truth is, people like to help because it makes them feel good, and I regret not asking. There are also 24-hour counselors available through the American Cancer Society. Knowing where my head was at throughout treatment, I should have definitely taken advantage of this service. The local Carol and Robert Wiseman Cancer Center also offers monthly support groups. After my great experience at the "Look Good, Feel Better" program, I did start attending their yoga classes on a regular basis, and it was the best thing I did for myself, but I could have done more. No one should go through this alone.

The last big piece of advice I would have for myself is to **embrace treatment**. I had resisted it every step of the way. I refused to call it chemo*therapy* because I felt that there was nothing therapeutic about it. I focused on the fact that I was having poison dripped through my veins. The truth is, I had agreed to drink the Kool-Aid, or in this case, drip it, and it would have been better for me to be 100% on board mentally. I did have fleeting moments of perspective after encounters with other patients, but they never lasted.

Interactions in the chemo room were a scarcity because most patients were infused with Benadryl as a part of their pre-meds and were therefore fast asleep. If a patient was awake, and not being dripped with A/C (which is easily identifiable because of its color, and signified a new case), it was for a good reason.

On the day that my sister accompanied me to The Big Chair, there was a young man about 30 years old and with a full head of hair seated in the recliner next to me. His young wife, perched on the stool in front of him, wept silently. In this close proximity, it was impossible not to overhear what was happening. He had been diagnosed just six weeks earlier with stage IV inoperable lung cancer. He had not come in for chemo because that was not an option for him. The cancer had already spread throughout his body. Instead, he was there because he had not eaten in four days, and could not keep down any liquids. They were giving him fluids, and then he was going to be admitted to the hospital next door. I was horrified and grateful at the same time as the nurse discussed hospice options with him. He did not have long to live.

On another occasion, I had arrived alone for my weekly follow-up appointment, and as I stepped off of the elevator, a bald young woman was being rushed out of the chemo room on a gurney. She was flanked by her middle aged parents. I don't know what the situation was, but the look on her mother's face was unmistakable. Once again, it hit home that I was one of the lucky ones.

On the day that I received my first infusion of Abraxane, there was an older woman sitting next to me with the same milky looking IV bag.

"What are you in for?" she asked, leaning in closer to me.

When I told her I had had stage II breast cancer, she looked perplexed.

"Hmm," she said. "I thought this cocktail was only reserved for people like me."

She went on to explain that she had stage IV inoperable pancreatic cancer, and was told in the beginning that she only had a year to live. She had been on Abraxane for 13 months, and was grateful that she had been able to enjoy one last Christmas with her children and grandchildren. She was now hoping to make it to Easter. Chemo for me was a poison to be dreaded and feared while for her it was an elixir of life.

"One holiday at a time," she said and smiled.

There was a man around my age that I saw in the chemo room frequently throughout the course of my treatment. He was hard to miss because he was wide awake, jovial, and always joking and flirting with the nurses. On several occasions I had the opportunity to sit near him and hear his story; the one that scared me the most. Four years earlier he had been diagnosed with stage III prostate cancer. Six months after his initial chemo treatment was completed, the cancer came back in his bones. He now had stage IV metastatic cancer, and had been on five different types of chemo over three years. The current cocktail that he was on was no longer working, and he would be switching to something else soon.

What struck me most about these encounters was the tranquility and grace that surrounded these amazing individuals who were fighting for just a little more time with their loved ones. In contrast, I was a spoiled brat. Embracing my time in Chemoland would have been a lot more productive and peaceful.

In the end, it is true. After this ordeal that I can only describe as life changing, I had become a lot stronger. I had also become one million times more compassionate, and one billion times more appreciative. Every day is a gift I will cherish.

Index

Resources

American Cancer Society – *offers a plethora of services including counseling, rides to treatment, the Look Good Feel Better program and access to local chapters that provide information, wigs, support, and more* www.cancer.org/ 800-227-2345

Breast Cancer Discussion Boards – *online support groups that are comprised of women in all different stages of treatment and recovery* www.community.breastcancer.org www.bcsupport.org www.inspire.com

Charity Organizations – *provides a list of organizations that offer financial assistance for cancer patients* www.managecancer.org

Chemo Angels – *a volunteer organization that offers support to cancer patients by sending "gifts of encouragement" throughout their journey* www.chemoangels.com

Cure Diva – *an online store that offers non-medical products for breast canter fighters, including head coverings, surgical bras, beauty products and more* www.curediva.com

Foods for Cancer – *provides nutritional guides and recipes for cancer patients* www.foodforbreatcancer.com www.cookforyourlife.org

National Cancer Legal Services Network – *an advocacy group that provides pro bono legal services for cancer patients* www.nclsn.org

Part Two
My Journal

July 15, 2013 – October 24, 2014

TAMZEN WHELAN

June 15:   *Noticed spotting in between menstrual cycles – mild concern Made appointment with GYN for pap smear to rule out cervical cancer*

July 8:   *Had appointment with GYN– he noticed a lump in my left breast – referred me to radiology for a transvaginal and bilateral ultrasound – mild concern*

July 19:   *Went for ultrasounds*

July 26:   *Saw midwife for results of ultrasounds – cyst in left breast of no concern – found several cysts in right breast – need to go back for a diagnostic mammogram – she thought it was just precautionary and nothing to worry about. Wasn't worried!*

July 29:   *Went for mammogram – new development in lymph node under right arm – went straight into another ultrasound – mild concern*

August 8:   *Saw the GYN for results of mammogram – lump in lymph node measures 1.5 centimeters – referred for biopsy – still mild concern – concern grows over the next week as I wait for the appointment and do some internet research – I may have lymphoma.*

August 20:   *I drive to appointment only to find out that it has been cancelled and that I actually wasn't scheduled for a biopsy – it was only a consultation
I am very upset and concern is growing – next appt. is in two days*

August 22:   *Dr. office calls to cancel appointment again. I break down and cry on the phone and tell her that she may as well order an autopsy rather than a biopsy – I call a different doctor and find a cancer patient advocate who calls the original office and gets me seen there that same day. Doctor L is great, and wants to do a biopsy right away, however is not available until next Tuesday. But he will come in especially to see me. My concern now is huge – what good is early detection if it is not followed by immediate treatment. It feels like the lump has grown to the size of an egg. Keep in mind that it didn't even show up on the ultrasound on July 19th.*

August 27:   *Day of biopsy – one hour before I have a full blown panic attack. I am dizzy, sweating profusely, and my torso is full of pain. I am convinced that the cancer has spread to all of my organs. I crawl outside and put 911 on speed dial, then call Jeff. We are considering that I should go to The Emergency room – then Dr. L's office calls and they want me to come in right away for the biopsy. I tell her about my pain, and she says to come in anyway if I can drive. I do. The nurse tells me that I cannot have my biopsy today because I can't sit still. Dr. L checks me out and finds nothing wrong. He insists on doing the biopsy. By the time he is done, the other pain is all but gone. I must wait one week for the results.*

August 30:   *I get a call from the Dr's office but no message. I am convinced that they want to see me right away because I am dying. I get a mild panic attack – light fever, increased heart rate. She calls back and tells me to come in on Tuesday at 9:00 am instead of 8:30. I am relieved. It will be a long weekend. I am hoping to have some fun in case it is the last time at least for a while. Three days to go… I am prepared for the worst which in my mind   is lymphoma. Anything else will be a relief.*

Later I find out that my medical is ending tomorrow… oh SHIT! Internet is down, so there is nothing I can do about it right now.

September 2:   *I was hoping to have some fun this weekend but I guess the stress got the better of me. Went to lunch in West Palm Beach on Saturday, but spent the Sunday and Monday in bed with vertigo trying not to think about cancer and no medical insurance. So happy that tomorrow is result day!! Think "benign"!!*

September 3:   *So relieved. Arrived at 9:00 am and only waited for about 5 minutes. Office lady called me up to inform me that my medical insurance was denied which I knew… Jeff came into the examining room with me. Doctor came in and said "It is not good." But what he didn't know was that his news was much better than where I had gone in my mind over the last three weeks! I have breast cancer. He said he believes it to be localized and that I will need a lumpectomy and radiation therapy. Once they do the lumpectomy, he can determine if the cancer has spread or not. If it has, they will need to remove lymph nodes and I may* need chemo. But as it stands, in the best case scenario, and I feel strongly that this is what it is...just the lumpectomy and radiation. I will not lose my hair!!! My relief is so great that I have so much energy and happiness today. Jeff and I went to breakfast after and for a swim in the ocean. I never knew that I would be so happy to hear the words "You have Breast Cancer."!!! Oh, the places our minds will take us...Biggest hurdle right now is getting my medical insurance taken care of.

September 4: Spent an hour on hold hoping to talk to a customer service agent about my medical insurance, but my call was never answered.

September 5: Called L's office at 11 am to touch base on appointments...went to voice mail. Anxiety is growing...early detection??????

September 6: Called L's office again in the am but went to voice mail. Called again at 2 pm but also went to voice mail. Called nurse Kristine, and she said "Angela" was working on it... Kristine calls back and asks me about insurance...I tell her I am working on it...she goes back to Angela's office and asks her...they want to know if I want to wait for my benefits...HELL NO! I tell her that it will be self pay if that is faster to get an appointment. She says yes and tells me that she or Angela will call me back about my appointment, which they insist must be with an oncologist before I can get surgery...They don't call...I call at 4:45 pm and I also have the number for the oncologist which I call but their office is closed…Angela calls FINALLY! Says that she has faxed my docs to the oncologist's office and that I should hear on Monday morning about my appointment with them…JESUS FUCKING CHRIST!!! When can I have this cancer taken out of me????

September 7: Had dinner with Kim and Chuck and Jonelle. Turns out a friend of Kim's, B, whom I met at Kim's and is my neighbor, is a pathologist at the hospital and knows my surgeon. She said she would look into my case! Nice relaxing evening.

September 8: Spoke with B on the phone in the morning. She was able to look up my chart and see that I have ductal cancer. The most common type. She was very supportive and said she would follow up tomorrow morning with L's office to get a date set for surgery. Feeling better! Great to have people supporting you…

September 9: B called and said she had spoken to L's office. They have my surgery earmarked for September 26. That seems very far away. She also called the oncologist and they told her that they would be calling me later today. They called a few hours later and set up an appointment for tomorrow morning. That's better!

September 10: Had a panic attack in the middle of the night, and Jeff said he would stay with me and go to my oncology appointment. Had a horrible panic attack on the way there. Threw up in the parking lot. They took my blood pressure which was 170 over 110. The nurse took it three times because she couldn't believe it. The oncologist was very supportive. I told about my growing fear because of the fact that the lump is now like an egg. She examined me and confirmed that it had doubled — now measuring 3 centimeters, but that didn't seem to worry her like it worries me. But of course it is not her body. However, because of my anxiety, she called Dr. L's office to see if she could move up my appointment for surgery. They did! It is now scheduled for September 18th! The reality is that that is when the real nightmare could actually just begin. She also said that people who smoke and go through radiation are twice as likely to develop lung cancer as those who just smoke. My last cigarette will be on September 17.

September 11: Spent two more hours on hold with the medical insurance. Went to visit the American Cancer Society, but it was just another cubbyhole with no answers — however, the very sweet girl told me that they have free wigs that I can borrow if I want. Yay me! For more pertinent information, I was told to call the hotline, which I did. The nice man was not much more helpful. I told him I wanted info on stress management, and quitting smoking. The only thing useful he gave me was a phone number to a patient advocate. I called them, and was told to wait 1 – 3 business days for a response.

The surgery center called and told me that I need to

come up with $3600 for the facility, and $437 for anesthesia prior to next Wednesday. Dr. L's office called and told me that I need to come up with $2600 by Friday to hold my appointment.

I try to take a nap but my mind keeps going to very dark places. I lay on the couch with the tv on, and that helps some. I feel very dizzy.

September 12: I take Maia to school early, and as soon as I get home to my empty house, a panic attack creeps up. I call Josh even though it is before 6 am in Seattle, and he talks me through it. Later the patient advocate calls. She is very gung ho, and believes that my insurance company dropping me is a crime. She tries to call them, but of course, like me, can't get through to a human.

I call Dr. L's office because my anxiety is building. The nurse tells me that he doesn't usually prescribe any medications, but when I tell her about my blood pressure, she gets me a prescription for Xanax.

I write an email to my mom and dad, asking for the money. I know they will help me, but it makes me feel worse to have to ask. Kathryn calls, and says she will call the office in the am to give a credit card number. I am relieved, but this is only the beginning.

The anesthesia department calls and I give them $437 from my debit card. Anxiety is building, but I am afraid of the Xanax, but by 7pm, I know I need to take one. I take one quarter, and it makes me feel so much better. Before bed, I take another half.

September 13: I slept so well! Too bad I had to get up at 7:30 to take Maia to school because I could have slept till noon. This is the first night I haven't woken up with an anxiety attack usually around 4 am. After I get home, I start calling the insurance company which is no walk in the park. I get the automated message to call back later 10 times, and finally get the message to press 1 to have someone call me back. They call back, and ask me to press 1 to speak with someone. When I press 1, an automated message says, "sorry, I don't understand. Goodbye!" I get this another 6 times. Finally, a real live person comes on the phone. My heart rate increases and I think I am going to have another panic attack. If I say the wrong thing, I am screwed. I don't say the wrong thing, and she tells me that there was an error and my medical coverage has been restored. It will be in the system by tomorrow morning!!!!! I cannot believe my ears. No copay, and full coverage!! I call the doctor's office, and they are willing to wait until Monday to run the insurance. I call the anesthesia department, and they are willing to refund my money on Monday after they run the insurance.

It is still early, and I have a great day. I get so much done, and do not have even one sign of a panic attack. I had no idea how much this issue was such a big part of my stress. I feel like everything is coming together, and it is all going to work out fine. Dr. L is going to remove this lump in five days, and I am going to need some radiation. End of nightmare!!! I will not allow myself to have any more dark thoughts. If they start, then Xanax!!

Going to have a good weekend. Planning a nice family day on Sunday, and then maybe I will go to the movies on Monday, and get a pedicure on Tuesday. Or a massage. Perfect start to the weekend!!

I feel like all of the obstacles have now disappeared…

September 14:   I call my family to let them know that my medical has been restored. Everyone is relieved. Jeff and I go get e cigarettes because the radiation oncologist said that a smoker who goes through radiation is twice as likely as a smoker to develop lung cancer.

September 15:   Had a great day with Maia and Jeff. We went to the Lion Safari in West Palm Beach. Very relaxing, but my inner dialogue would not shut up anyway. "I am going to die because of the signs such as…." "I am not going to die because of the signs such as…" torture!! B called to invite us over for coffee at 8 pm. I let her know that we are having a family day because surgery has been pushed up for this Wednesday.

September 16:   Jeff went to work and Maia went to school. I hate to be alone… Made all the calls I needed to in order to let everyone (providers) know that my insurance has been restored. Two more days until surgery. It is still early so I put on the TV and try to take a nap. Mild panic attack. So happy to pick Maia up and take the dogs for a walk. I never have a panic attack when I am with Maia. She still has not told her friends....We get a pedicure and go for a nice walk with the dogs. I am in a really good mental space and am thinking very positive thoughts. My mom calls and starts crying on the phone. I am pissed...I don't need to think about dying right now.

September 17: One day to go! My worst fear is that they are going to call and cancel my surgery for tomorrow. I go shopping and cook casseroles so that Maia and Jeff will have food while I am down after surgery. I am thinking about how they will get along if I die. I get kind messages from Kim, Jonelle, and Aaron. I get an email form Linda saying that she will be in Ft Lauderdale in October, so I let her know that I have breast cancer and probably wont be able to meet her....get a text from her and Ilsa! Guess I forgot cancer protocol and have worried them...can't deal with them tonight. I think positive thoughts, and fight back the negative ones. I visualize myself walking into the surgery center, calm and non-fearing. Can't eat (don't care) or drink anything after midnight. Surgery is at 1 pm – check in at 12 pm – so I can drink water at 7 am tomorrow morning. I set my alarm and hope I can sleep. I haven't slept past 5 am for weeks. I drink lots of wine and one bottle of water at midnight.

September 18: I wake up at 5 am as usual and drink some water. I try to get back to sleep but toss and turn until my water alarm goes off at 7 am. I drink the full 16 ounces. I lay back down but cannot sleep. I get up at 9 am and dry heave. At least I know my stomach is empty and they won't refuse surgery!! I toss and turn more so Jeff says we should get something done. I don't want to but I know he is right. We take my car in and stop by Petsmart. They won't give me any antibiotics for Kai because it has been too long (his skin infection is back and I have been ignoring it). We go home and wait. I dry heave some more, and we leave at 11:20. We arrive at the surgery center at 11:45 and they are ready for me. They tell me that they will prep me and that Jeff can come back and see me before Dr. L arrives.

My IV goes in and I meet the anesthesiologist. I am so relieved that he is a man, and no chance it is my crazy neighbor lady. I tell him about my loose crown, and he assures me that he will stay with me and monitor me the entire time.

My blood pressure is sky high, so the nurse goes to get Jeff to calm me down. Some how he makes me laugh, and I get on an even keel. I don't want anything to stop me from having this surgery even though I am scared.

Soon the nurse is back and bumps up my IV to something stronger – it is time for the injection *through my nipple so that they can see if the cancer has spread to my lymph nodes. I am feeling pretty good, like I had about five margaritas. They say it's time, and Jeff has to go... They wheel me off to the operating room, and the last thing I remember is about six to eight people standing around me. They ask me to slide over onto a table under six huge spot lights.*

The next thing I know, I wake up in the recovery room. I am very cold and shaking. I ask for Jeff, but they won't let him in yet. It is 3:15. I don't know how long I have been out, but I know that surgery started at around 1:30. I can't gauge if this good or bad.

Finally Jeff comes in. He tells me that it is all good. I don't know what that means. Then he tells me that they didn't find anything in my lymph nodes. I had forgotten to worry about that, but now I am elated! The doctor comes in and seems relieved as well.

We leave the hospital at about 4 pm, and I text Maia to let her know to send her boyfriend home. I text all of my family and friends to let them know the good news. We get home, and I go get in bed. I feel so happy and relieved. Jeff cooks dinner, and we all watch the X Factor. It almost feels like normal. We are all in excellent spirits. I can't imagine how the night would have gone if the news hadn't been the best possible.

I am hoping for a great night sleep, but this isn't possible. I refuse to take the pain killers, and my breast aches. But the bigger problem is that I cannot roll over. None of it matters. I feel I am cancer free!!!!

September 20: The last two days have been a big movie marathon. Jeff has been with me, cooking and attending to my every need. I have a drain hanging from a tube outside my breast that needs to be cleared every four hours or so. It is pinned to my bra and very annoying! I can't take a shower, but we are still so happy that the results were good. I get several bunches of flowers delivered and my family and friends have been texting and calling. Everyone is so relieved and surprised. I feel good. Tired, and achy, and dirty, but good.

September 22: Jeff and I go to the mall to get haircuts. My main motivation is to get my hair washed!! Then we go to the store for food. I am exhausted and must take a nap. Jeff makes dinner as usual, and he and Maia take the dogs out.

September 23: It's Monday, and I call L's office to see if I can get my drain out. I go in at 1:30 and have it removed. I go home and take my first shower since the surgery last Wednesday. Feeling better! I am able to cook dinner and take the dogs out for a walk.

September 26: I have my post op appointment with L. He says that everything is out, but because I have a very aggressive type of cancer, I must have chemotherapy. I am not panicked. But I don't want to lose my hair. Guess I don't have a choice. I call Kim, and she says her treatment lasted six months. Yuk... Wigs for Christmas? She sent me pictures of herself bald, and she actually looked pretty good. She preferred bandanas and hats. I have an appointment with the chemo witch doctors on Monday. I guess this is going to happen pretty soon...

September 30: Had oncology appointment. Totally panicked... heart rate was 167/120. He prescribed valium which I don't want to take... said chemo was necessary. 1 out of 3 women that have had my type of cancer die if they don't go to chemo. Have to have an EKG to make sure my heart can handle chemo...fuck. With all of my panic attacks, I am worried about my heart, but if it is weak, at least I will avoid chemo! I also must have a port installed for IV's. I don't want it. Makes me feel like a sickly patient...

October 1: Oncologist office calls... must also have a PET scan because one of my blood tests revealed that I may have cancer elsewhere... I am totally freaked. Kim texts me and says that she had one also but it was precautionary. This doesn't sound precautionary to me... I try to reason this out... if I have another type of cancer, like leukemia, I am destined to die... chances are slim that I have two cancers at the same time... I am still freaked...

October 2:   *Woke up worried, and cancelled my dentist appointment. Couldn't face Lisa and Cindy and tell them that I have breast cancer. I told Lisa on the phone, and she was very supportive. Told Lisa that the next time she saw me, I would be bald. She said that I would still be beautiful... Went for EKG. Had a panic attack at lunch with Jeff before. Worried that my heart isn't strong enough. We went to the beach after lunch, which was relaxing, and then to the hospital. They would not let Jeff into the room with me, which turned out to be someone's office with a couple of tables in it set up for EKG's. They put me on the table and injected me with something I'm sure was radioactive, and then plugged me in. The machine made a buzz, and they said not to worry. They wiped me down, and continued to connect me. Finally succeeding, but not before I was freaked out. Then the tunnel enclosed me, but there were windows on the side so I could see out. Then the camera came down, and they said that each picture would take 10 minutes. I could feel the whoosh as my blood and heart beat did there thing, and kept repeating to myself that I was in the safest place if I was going to have a heart attack. The phone kept ringing, and the staff was not concerned with me whatsoever. Finally, after way after 10 minutes on the second picture, they said I was done...*

October 3:   *Jeff went to work, so I am on my own. I am not in a good frame of mind at all. Don't know if I am going to hear that my heart is not good, or if I may have* more cancer… *very scared for the scan next Wednesday. The phone rings, and I cannot answer it. I cannot have any more bad news today. I don't think I can handle it alone. I let it go to voice mail but can't even check it. Instead I drive to the book store, and distract myself looking at books that I will need in the coming weeks. I finally build up the confidence to listen to my voice mail in the non-fiction isle. It is the Vet calling for a follow up appointment with Kai. I am soooo relieved. The call also came in at 11:11 which it seems is always the time that I look at the clock lately. 11:11 can no longer scare me.*

October 5:   *Maia and I go shopping for birthday presents for her friends and homecoming shoes. We are mostly successful, and I have a good day with my daughter. Jeff and I have dinner with Aaron and Jonelle. We have a good time, and they are both very supportive. Aaron is confident that I will breeze through this because my lymph nodes are clear. He also tells me that after chemo, I will feel like I have the flu a few days later, lasting for a few days, but nothing drastic. Jonelle offers to go have fun with me when I feel up to it. This was a very good day! Portal goes in on Monday, and I will do my best not to worry about that, or the scan on Wednesday that may reveal more cancer.*

October 7:   *Portal goes in without a problem. Even harder to sleep now with surgeries on both sides. Jeff is home with me all day but has to go to work tomorrow.*

October 9: PET scan day – I think I will have to take a valium for this but I end up not. I am so tired, that I am pretty much zonked out by the time the technologist puts me in the room and injects me the radioactivity. I have to stay in the room alone for one hour. I sit back and relax, knowing that Jeff is just on the other side of the door. After an hour, I go into the scanning machine. It slides me in and out taking pictures, and then takes 5 pictures starting with my head. Each picture is supposed to be 3 minutes but it feels longer than that. At first, I feel very claustrophobic, but once my head is out it is ok. It is very hard to stay still. When I am done, the technician says he thinks it is very "optimistic" but I won't get the results until Monday – THE BIG DAY...chemo begins...

October 11: I am feeling pretty well recovered from Monday's surgery. Was able to take both dogs for a walk by myself. Called Kim to ask her what a "bad" day was like. She said that some days she could only stay in bed and stare at the ceiling...but they weren't all like that. She also took her kids to school and made dinner. She was able to walk up her hill many days, but didn't have the energy to run. If my PET scan is negative, I will embrace chemo. It is supposed to save my life after all!!! Three days to go...

October 14: First day of chemo. Couldn't sleep last night thinking of all that might go wrong. Have to keep reminding myself that chemo is a treatment even *though it feels like a 6 month prison sentence. Got to the Dr.'s office at 9:45. Had just enough time to get my heart rate good and freaked out. Jeff was there to steady me. The good news is that my PET scan came back clean, and then I had to resign myself to the fact that there is no way out – I must do chemo.*

I have been sitting in the chemo chair for about 2 hours now. They started off slowly, using my port for the first time with an anti-nausea drip, then we moved on to the first round of chemo which was bright red. I started feeling light headed but I'm pretty sure that was just psychological. I went to the bathroom with my IV – and as expected, my pee is pink. I am now on my second bag of chemo. The room is pleasant. I have a view of the Indian River and some patients are chatting. Others are reading and most are sleeping. It's weird to be sitting here, but I suppose it's true that a person can get used to anything. I'm nervous for the week ahead, to see how my body reacts, but I can/will endure. Should be bald around Halloween!!! By the time we got home, it was 4 pm. Took a nap, and spent the rest of the evening on the couch – very tired and legs feel very heavy. It got better by bedtime.

October 15: *I did not sleep well at all. Most likely because I didn't have any wine. Slept from 12 am – 2:30 and lay awake the rest of the night thinking about aneurisms because I had a pounding headache. Chemo can't be good for the brain! I got up at 7:30 and ate an egg and cranberry juice – then took my* anti-nausea medicine. Jeff and Maia left at 8:30 and I was able to sleep until 11:30. Was still tired so had a cup of soup and stayed in bed watching TV and trying to sleep until 2 pm. Took a shower and went to the doctor for my shot of white blood cell boost. The nurse said that I would have severe bone pain in about two hours, and lasting for about 2 hours, but in the long run it would make me feel better. Went to Luna's for a slice of pizza – ate the whole thing (worried because I weigh 123 lbs. I don't want to get so I am sickly looking). Picked Maia up at 4 pm and we went fundraising. Felt like I was racing against the clock – wanted to get home before I was in pain. Got home by 5 pm – legs feel like fire – but not really horrible. Maia will have to walk the dogs by herself today : (

October 16:   Got up and thought I was feeling great, but after a few minutes on my feet, realized that I needed to get back to bed – low energy and heavy/tingling feeling in my legs. Ate a piece of toast and drank cranberry juice then took a nausea pill. Called the nurse and left a message because I have not had a bowel movement since I think Sunday, the day before chemo. Spent the day in bed watching TV and reading – waiting for the nurse to call. Got up at 2 pm, took a shower and went to meet Maia at CVS. Picked up some meds, but missed the call from the nurse. Finally got her on the phone, and she said not to take what I had bought. Took Maia to the gym, and went to the market for dinner and the correct meds. Took Milk of Magnesia at 5:30 pm – ate black bean chili at 9 pm, and still haven't pooped. Just took one of the other pills that is supposed to work overnight (Senekot-S). It is now 10:30, and I am in bed and I still haven't pooped. Tomorrow could be a great day, or a horrible one.....

October 17: Woke up at 5 am and took more Milk of Magnesia...still no action. Maia woke me up at 8 am and still nothing. I made a cup of green tea and a bowl of grapes, and sat in bed reading until...finally at 9:30 am it worked!! I read for a while longer and then slept until 11:30. Had lunch and read/slept/watched TV until 2 pm then got ready to pick up Maia. The BIG BAD never came! Managed to take Maia to the gym and then back to school for the homecoming parade, and even cooked dinner. The heaviness in my legs seems to be subsiding. I was able to take the dogs on the mailbox run last night and tonight. Seems like the worst day was the first, not 3 days later like everyone said – I hope that is a good sign and I don't get slammed with the next round...

October 20: Friday was a good day and I thought that I had sailed through the week. Ran errands from about 3 – 6:30, taking Maia around – I felt almost normal! Then, when I tried to make dinner around 8 pm, I was slammed hard. Heart palpitations, extreme dizziness – couldn't stand up. Maybe I over did it during the day – I even cleaned the house! Jeff had to make dinner – I still had an appetite, but could barely walk to bed.

Slept till 11:30 on Saturday – still feeling dizzy and off balance. Couldn't walk around. Jeff ordered Chinese for dinner and we watched movies. Did nothing productive at all. This am I woke up at 9 am to Jeff bringing me a muffin. Felt a little better – not so off balance – but became constipated again. More Milk of Magnesia for me…Napped and then ran errands w/Maia – feeling much better – only slightly off balance. Went out for milkshakes and fries!! Can't remember the last time I had a milkshake – maybe 5 years ago. It's been over a week since I've had any wine or a cigarette. You'd think I'd be feeling like a million dollars! Can I really take 5 months of this? Can Jeff and Maia? It's only been one week!!

October 21: *Had a good day. Slept/read/ate until 1 pm then went to the Dr. for blood work. Low white cell count – to be expected – stay away from public places and sick people. Was able to run some errands and pick Maia up at 3 pm – then we took the dogs to Haney – my first real walk in over a week. Took Maia to the gym then rested until I picked her up. Made her dinner and then rested again. Tried to make dinner around 8 pm, but got dizzy. I guess I am not back to normal after all – Jeff and I got into a fight over making dinner and I had an emotional break down. Perhaps I really need to rethink 5 months of chemo…Is it worth 8 % points? I am a prisoner of my own body.*

October 22: *Had a great day!! OK – it's all relative. Met Kim for* *breakfast at the Blue Door, and then went to Bathtub Beach for a walk/swim. Had a very nice time. Kim leaves for San Fran next week – I'm really going to miss her. Got home and had a nap then shower and went to pick Maia up and went to Target. Got a calorie boosting vanilla been frapaccino. I'm down to 120 lbs and DO NOT want to lose any more – at least not this way. I rested for a bit when we got home, then made dinner early – watched TV and ate w/Maia until now (9 pm). I feel like I need to pack productivity in over the next few days while I am still feeling good. Can't wait to fast forward 5 months and remember what it actually means to feel good!!*

October 23: *Had a good day – wish every day could stay just like this one for the next five months. I got Betsy a plane ticket out!! So excited for her to come…just wish it was going to be more fun. I will be bald when she gets here. I was able to take the dogs out today and run errands, and make dinner. I never even got dizzy. Though I did take a hard nap from 5 – 5:30 pm. I am really dreading Monday and having to go through this cycle again over the next two weeks. When this is all over, I want to: play tennis, go to The Keys, finish my first book (maybe sooner), take photography (maybe sooner), try windsurfing, explore more places…LIVE!!!*

October 24: *Had a very productive day. Got up at 10 am and started hitting my To Do List – got about half way through by 2 pm – then I got ready and picked up*

Maia w/the dogs. We took them to the beach for a nice walk then we went and got our nails done! After that, I made dinner and we watched "Little Miss Sunshine" – good for a laugh. I haven't napped all day and I ALMOST feel normal. In bed now at 9:30. I am feeling so frustrated that I have to go back on Monday and watch the poison that I going to make me sick all next week, drip into my veins. That seems insane! Ah...but I am committed – I have about one week left w/my hair. Going to order head scarves tomorrow. Three days left to be normal for another week...

October 25: *My hair started falling out today. I ordered a few head scarves and then I got a wig in the mail from Josh! I will need to cut my hair this weekend – in stages – down to a buzz cut. I guess there is no backing out now! I felt about 90% normal today. Only two days left of normalcy. Got a nice edible bouquet of fruit from friends in LA. It would have been easier to go through this in LA where I actually had a group of friends. All of my friends here are gone. Oh, well. Betsy is coming in November and Josh in December. Kathryn is ready to come too if I need her. I have a lot to do this weekend but will try to enjoy every minute of it. We will do our traditional pumpkin carving on Saturday.*

October 27: *Yesterday I had Maia cut my hair up to my shoulders. Then last night I had two glasses of wine for the first time in two weeks! My hair continues to fall out, but none of the scarves have arrived that are* *supposed to cover my head. I think I will have Jeff give me a buzz cut tomorrow afternoon anyway. We carved pumpkins tonight and I am feeling just a hair shy of 100%. I am dreading the week to come so much. I do not want to sit in that chair tomorrow morning and watch the poison drip into my veins – this past week has been so good, and this coming week will probably be worse than the first week. . .2 weeks down – 18 to go!*

October 28:   *Week 3 – second round of chemo today. Dr. was running behind so we didn't finish until after 2 pm – then had lunch and picked up Maia. Home around 3:15 and nap until 4:30. I was leaving a hair trail all around today, so I had Jeff buzz off the remainder this afternoon. It is about a ½ inch with several bald spots. Luckily, all of the head covers arrived today, so I have been trying them out. Had dinner around 8 pm and watched the Seahawk game. I feel a little bit tired and tingly, but not as bad as I did on Monday in week 1. I have a new plan of attack this week – no cooking, dinner by 7 pm and off my feet by 7 pm and plenty of rest during the day. Hoping for an uneventful, smooth week.*

October 29:   *Had trouble sleeping last night. My heart sounded so loud it kept me up. I had maybe 5 hours of sleep. Went in this afternoon for the white cell boost – was told it is cumulative but I only got a mild tingling this time. I felt pretty good all day, just tired. I talked to the nurse about heart palpitations, and she didn't have much to offer except to see my* cardiologist (which I don't have), and to talk to the oncologist on Monday when I go for my blood test. I feel tense, so perhaps it is just stress induced. I have a slight fever of 99.4. Hopefully I will have a good night sleep and not feel bad tomorrow...

October 30: I had a horrible night sleep – heart palpitations – slept maybe 4 hours. Ironically, I felt great today except for lack of sleep. No dizziness, no heavy limbs, nothing weird. I called the nurse and she still didn't have an answer for my heart, but she said to stop taking the steroid pill in the morning that goes along with the anti-nausea medicine and that may help. I didn't realize it was a steroid I had been taking. She also said it could be from the white cell boost. It is 8:30 and I am already in bed. If I can't sleep, I will take a ¼ valium. I am sleep deprived. If I sleep tonight, I will feel good tomorrow – it's Halloween!

October 31: I finally slept, and when I woke up at 8 am I felt pretty good, but went back to sleep and at 9:30 the chemo fog arrived. Been in bed all day feeling like shit. It's worse than the flu because I really feel like I am in a chemical fog. Add heart palpitations, and oh, boy, it's a regular party with no sleep! I ordered a pizza for dinner, and Jeff handled the door for trick-or-treaters by himself. I couldn't get off the couch. I have pain in all of my joints and bones. Maia is off celebrating Halloween with her friends, so the dogs didn't get a walk. Happy fricken Halloween. Chemo sucks! And who knows what tomorrow has in store *for me. Oh, and got my period today. Yay me.*

November 1: *Today was much like yesterday. I was unable to get out of bed accept to quickly grab food and go to the bathroom. I feel totally off balance if I stand more than a few minutes. The poor dogs didn't get outside until Maia came home at 4 pm. I hope I wake up tomorrow morning and the fog has lifted. I would love to have a solid week to feel good. Betsy comes on Tuesday. I hope she is up to dealing with this/me – and all of my paranoia! It is 10 pm, and I am in bed waiting for Maia to get home and then I will turn out the light and get a great sleep and wake up to a fresh new day.*

November 2: *Another lost day. Feeling better but still no energy to get out of bed. Spent the day reading, watching TV and sleeping while Jeff did my job of driving Maia around. Started getting heart palpitations after dinner which escalated into a panic attack, so I took a ¼ xanax. It helped but I really do not want to live with these heart issues. It really scares me. I will talk to the Dr. on Monday when I go in for my blood test. I am really hoping that I will wake up tomorrow feeling well enough to get out of the house – get to the store and take the dogs out, and be able to do laundry and get ready for Betsy. I also hope for a good night sleep.*

November 3: *Another day in bed. My heart was fluttering on and off all day. By 6 pm it finally felt like I had a breakthrough to the other side. Feeling MUCH* better. Jeff made a big dinner and I moved to the couch for the Seahawks game. I have been drinking crazy amounts of water and will ask about diabetes tomorrow morning when I go in for my blood test. Hopefully the Dr. will be able to see me. I did a lot more research on the type of cancer that I had, and it is mow more clear to me that even though there is only a 20% chance that it will come back, I should go through with the chemo because it can come back in other parts of the body where it wouldn't be so easily detected. I hope the doc can solve the heart palpitation issue (my biggest complaint).

November 4: Week 4 – Went in for blood test this am. Had a pull blown panic attack in the office – did not see it coming. In the end, Dr. said that my issues of weight loss (down to 118 lbs) and hunger/thirst and increased heart rate could all be a side effect of the steroids that go with the anti-nausea meds. I don't have diabetes and it will go away. He asked if I had been taking the Valium, and when I said no, he gave me a prescription for Ativan in the hopes that I will actually take it. I will, but hopefully won't need it this week. I am feeling so much better today. Did some cleaning to get ready for Betsy and ran some errands. Betsy will be here tomorrow night!! Can't wait to see her and am so relieved that I am feeling good – ready for a good week! Hoping to go to the movies and the beach and to get my wig a haircut! I still haven't lost my eyebrows.

November 5: Had a GREAT day! Got up at 9 am and hit my To

Do list. Took a few breaks but did not nap at all. Went for a milkshake in the afternoon – trying to build my weight back up before the next round of chemo. Then Maia and I took the dogs for a nice walk. Got home around 6 pm and started dinner. Jeff arrived with Betsy around 8 pm and we all had dinner together, then talked and watched TV. It is now 11 pm and I am still feeling good! Got a care package in the mail from more LA friends – very sweet. All of my friends have been so supportive, sending me texts and facebook messages weekly. I'm looking forward to the next few good days with my sister.

November 6: Busiest day I have had yet – though not really busy by normal standards. I made a crock pot dinner this am and then B and I went shopping, to lunch, and to the supermarket. Took a one hour break and B and Maia went to the gym. I really wish that I could have gone, too, but my energy was waning, so I stayed home and read. They got back around 6 pm, and we had dinner and watched the X factor. I am now in bed at 10:30 pm. B is going to the gym in the morning, and then we are going to downtown Stuart to find Florida souvenirs. I never ever want to go back to chemo again! Maybe it won't be so bad next week. This week (week 4) has been better than week 2.

November 7: Very disappointing day. Woke up at 8 am feeling very dizzy. All of our plans couldn't happen – I had to stay in bed all day. B went to the store, and the *gym, and to pick up Maia without me. I tried to take a shower in the afternoon, but got really dizzy and I had to call out for B to help me back to bed. I just drank 10 bottles of water and finally feel better at 10 pm. I think I over did it yesterday, and then had the sugary Starbucks drink and didn't drink enough water, so I was extremely dehydrated. I WANT MY DAY BACK! Tomorrow we are going to the beach — if I am feeling well, and if the weather is good. Maia is out of school so it will be the three of us. I really want a good day.*

November 8: *Good day! Went with B and Maia and walked around downtown Stuart. Went to a hair salon and got my wig a haircut. Wore it out to lunch, then came back and had a nap. B and Maia took the dogs out in the rain. B made dinner, and Maia's friends came for a sleepover. The first sleepover since August when this nightmare began. We ran into one of her friends downtown, and she saw me wearing a head scarf for the first time and could barely look at me. I guess it's weird for other people to see me without hair. I started having mild heart palpitations this evening and can't understand why, but took ½ an Ativan and they went away. Was able to take the dogs out for a pm walk. Now in bed at 11 pm.*

November 9: *Had a nice family day — went to the movies. Never mind that we saw "Gravity" and I had to keep my eyes closed throughout 90% of the movie! I wore my wig as "Claire". Ate popcorn and had a little soda. Soda doesn't taste the same on chemo. We had a nice* dinner, and I enjoyed two glasses of wine. I am drinking extra water to make up for it, which is hard because I already had 12 bottles today. The last thing I want is to get dehydrated again. I would love to get one more day of normalcy before chemo on Monday. I am so glad that my sister is here to help me through next week. I feel bad that she has to live my pathetic life these two weeks – but I am grateful. In bed now at 11 pm. Hoping for good weather for a beach day tomorrow.

November 10: Good day. B and I went to Bathtub Beach. It was too rough to go in all the way, but I was able to get wet. We sat in the sun for about a half hour then went grocery shopping and got home around 3 pm. I rested until about 5 pm, and then we made ribs. It's 10:30 and I am ready for bed, but not for tomorrow. If the Dr. won't lighten up on the steroids at least, I don't think I can go through with it. I can't handle another week of sleepless nights, heart palpitations, and turning into a bag of bones – not to mention drowning myself in 12 bottles of water every day. He can't possibly think that is healthy!

November 11: Start of week 5 – 3rd AC treatment. I slept in/stayed in bed feeling depressed that I have to go to chemo today. Was happy that my appointment was changed to later in the day. I didn't have to rush and was able to eat a full sandwich before. Betsy came with me today. I was nervous about talking to Dr. Dracula and my blood pressure was high – but in the end, he agreed to cut down my steroid, and I am not *going in for the white blood cell boost tomorrow because I told him about feeling dizzy/off balance, and that I think that is the cause. Instead I go next week to monitor my white blood cell count and may get a milder dose if I need it. B and I are going to work hard to get the count up naturally over this next week with food! Dr. also wants me to go for an MRI, but I told the front desk scheduler girl to hold off until I get through this week. If I don't experience that intense dizzy/off balance nightmare, then it was the shot. If I do, then it could be the chemo. He wanted to rule out brain cancer, but I am not interested in staying in a tube for an hour when obviously something I am being given is causing the dizziness. He shook his head at me in disapproval as I was leaving. Oh well. When I got home, my limbs became heavy and tingly and my heart rate increased. I started to feel slightly light headed until I ate dinner. Took an Ativan and am in bed at 9:30. Hoping for an easier ride this week. The other nice thing is that I don't have to go back to chemo for 3 weeks — until my white blood cell count is acceptable. That means I can enjoy Thanksgiving!!*

November 12: *I didn't get much sleep last night — was afraid to go to sleep because I was worried that I would never wake up. Sounds silly, but the thing with cancer (or any other deadly disease I suppose), is that the weight of it never leaves you. I wake up with it heavy on my mind, and it lingers on my brain all day and through the night. Funny I have not had one dream that I recall except for having sand packed in*

my mouth and waking up needing 3 bottles of water.
I stayed in bed most of the day – trying to sleep, but
more reading and searching the internet for the side
effects of all the meds I have suddenly found myself
on. Got up around 2 pm, ate did some light (very)
cleaning and then B and I took the dogs out and
picked up Maia at 5 pm. B made an awesome salmon
dinner with all the ingredients to help fuel my white
blood dell count. I didn't have the booster shot
today, so I am feeling pretty good! Just mildly
fatigued. I am really hoping that the rest of the week
will go much better now that I don't have the added
steroid or the booster. Hopefully I won't be dizzy or
off balance and can avoid the dreaded MRI because
I do not have an effing brain tumor. Hopefully,
hopefully, hopefully, it was a side effect of the shot
– and not the chemo. The next few days should tell.
One funny side effect I experienced today that was
new to me was a flushed face. It looked like I had a
sunburn. The family said I looked better with it!
Maybe I am going through early menopause – a
possible side effect of chemo. I still have my eyebrows
and lashes!

November 13:   The chemo fog rolled in at about 11 am. Got the
tingling in limbs and general groggy, foggy feeling all
over. The worst of it lasted until around 3 pm. I did
not get slammed with the dizzy/off balance ordeal
and am really hoping that it won't hit tomorrow.
It's 10:30 and I'm in bed feeling just ok.

November 14:   Another day much like yesterday without the fog – a

*big improvement over week 3, but still in bed all day.
B took Maia to her National Honor Society
Induction and parent night for driver's Ed. I stayed
home and took a bath. In bed now at 10:30. I am
really feeling so over this. The stress, the fatigue, the
what-ifs, the unpredictable side effects. I just want
to get back to normal. March feels like a very, very
long time away…Hopefully tomorrow I will at least
be able to get out of the house.*

November 15: *I am having a much faster recovery this week. I was
able to run a few errands w/B today, then took a
rest, and drove Maia to her friend's house. Then
dinner and TV. Now at 10 pm I am in bed. Was
unable to take the dogs out, but this is a huge
improvement over week 3! Just hoping I can get my
white blood cells up. Betsy leaves on Tuesday – only
three more days. It's going to be difficult without her
not only because she has been doing all the cooking
and cleaning, but because she brings the household
energy up. And I will be alone for the most part.*

November 16: *Stayed in bed most of the day – got up around 2 pm –
showered, went to the store w/B. Feeling better than
yesterday but still too tired to do much. I did have a
drink after dinner while we watched a movie –
something I normally don't do on a chemo week, so I
guess this week really was much better. I am hoping
that I will feel strong enough to get out and enjoy the
nice weather tomorrow – maybe go to the beach. I
still have two entire weeks before chemo again!!
Hopefully I can be productive. I will be so sorry to*

see Betsy leave. Only 4 months to go!! Ha ha.

November 17: Very good day! B and I went to the beach. It was a beautiful day – warm and breezy. The water was a tad cold, but felt great! Then we picked Maia up and went grocery shopping. I took a nap from 4 – 5 while B and Maia went to the gym and then walked the dogs. Jeff and I made dinner – gave B the night off. I am now in bed at 10 pm exhausted but feeling good. Tomorrow we go see what my white blood cell count reads. Hopefully all the "right" foods we ate this week will have paid off. I need to avoid that shot. In any case, I will not accept it tomorrow. Last day for B to be here☹

November 18: I was very tired today. Had to go to the doc at 2 pm for a blood test, and the pre-anxiety set in around noon. By the time we got to the office my blood pressure was sky high. The nurse congratulated me on my blood counts, though they don't look much different to me from before. But as long as I avoid the shot, whatever! We stopped by the resource center and I met the social worker and coordinator and they suggested I come to a support group. I didn't think I would be interested because I don't want to sit around and hear a bunch of whining, but they told me that the group also does meditation and yoga. That could be fun! Anyway, I will give it a try. Betsy leaves tomorrow morning. I am sad to see her go, but Josh is coming for Christmas so I have another sibling to look forward to! Earlier today, I noticed dark spots on my temples and cheeks – I had the nurse look at it but she didn't think it was anything. However, any changes to my body make me alarmed. I always think "what now?"! The next couple of weeks will be good ones!

November 19: B left early this morning. A long day of traveling for her. I had a good day. Took the dogs for a walk at the bridge, had a nice nap and then took Maia to her dermatology appointment. We didn't get home until 6:30. One of Jeff's co-workers sent dinner home for us. Very sweet! Tomorrow I need to get to the store for some healthy cell boosting food since I lost my cook and nursemaid! I am feeling very good. I read that you shouldn't totally give in to the fatigue – exercise will help and naps should be no more than 45 minutes. Am going to make an appointment with a nutritionist tomorrow.

November 20: I truly feel almost effing normal! So much so that I double dread having another treatment!! Doesn't that word imply that I am supposed to feel good after? Anyway, I felt quite productive today. Did the grocery shopping, picked up the kid, did some cleaning, took the dogs for a walk, cooked dinner three times, took Maia to a study group at Barnes and Noble, made some phone calls... but now exhausted at 10 pm. Have to get up at 9 am tomorrow to go to the dentist, and am looking forward to another productive day! I still have a week and a half!!

November 21: Can't catch a break! Went to the dentist today to find out that I indeed have an infection (It woke me up last night – pain and sweats). He wants to pull it and prep it for an implant, but I am not sure if that is allowed. I called the oncologist's office and they got my some super strand of antibiotics that are supposed to give me indigestion and diarrhea. Yay me! I have been sporting a fever of around 99 all evening. What I don't know is if I can get the tooth pulled or if this will delay my next "treatment" - just hoping my fever won't spike and land me in the hospital. I ask again… is all this really worth it??

November 22: So the antibiotics make my heart beat fast – go figure. Seems like everything I take these days has that effect. Lucky me! I am not taking the third dose tonight. Checked my blood pressure at the store today – 115/70 – last week it was 120/80. It doesn't seem high to warrant the high blood pressure medicine, but perhaps I am wrong. Not feeling good today, but at least I don't have a fever. Not a very productive day. Rest seems like the best cure for a rapid heart beat. I WANT MY LIFE BACK!!!!

November 23: Today was pretty messed up. I couldn't sleep last night. Finally got to sleep around 1:30 am but woke up at 4 am with a nightmare. Got back to sleep around 5:30 and slept till 7:30. Researched the side effects of the antibiotic versus the chance of a spreading mouth infection, so I could decide whether or not to take them. In the end, I chose not to. Took an afternoon nap and read the rest of the day. My fever came on about 5 pm at 99.6. I took Tylenol around 8 pm which knocked it back down. It is not 11:30 and I am tired but as usual, afraid to go to sleep. This is a messed up world to live in (Chemoland). And this was supposed to be a great week...

November 24: More of the same – fever hit an all time high of 100.6 this afternoon. I decided to go back to the dreaded antibiotics and just stay in bed. It has worked out just fine. Tylenol takes the fever down. Just took the second pill of the day (now at 10 pm). Now I wish I had just followed through yesterday – oh hindsight! I see my oncologist tomorrow at 2 pm. Then we can decide what to do about the tooth. Good thing I don't have chemo tomorrow. No way I could do it in this condition anyway. Jeff and Maia have been so sweet and helpful – going to the store, cooking, walking the dogs, getting me water and food...Thank God for them!!

November 25: Another messed up day. Fever hit 101 last night. In bed all day until Dr. appointment at 2 pm. They took a lot of blood and gave me the lighter white blood cell boost. Hopefully that along with the antibiotics will take down my fever soon, like by tomorrow! I am so sick of all this bullshit. Dr. said to go to the ER if I get the chills/shakes. Great. Don't think I will get any sleep tonight.

November 26: The day got off to a slow start, but I am feeling sooo much better. My fever has not gone above 99.6 and I was able to take the dogs out and help with dinner.

Went to the Dr. this afternoon for another white cell boost – this version is a huge improvement. My body still gets a little off balance, but NOTHING compared to my reaction to the Neulasta. Had a wake up call – a friend who lost his wife to breast cancer 5 years ago posted that that he was going out to celebrate her life tonight. She would have been 52. I am in good shape here, and should be more embracing of my treatment. I'm sure she would have been beyond ecstatic to be in my position. Gotta keep it in perspective. Tomorrow morning I go get my blood checked to see if my white cell count is high enough to get my tooth pulled. I kind of hope it isn't so I can thoroughly enjoy the next 5 days!

November 27:   *NO MORE FEVER!! Got my white blood cell count this morning – it was way high at 15%! Then on to have my tooth pulled. I am feeling so much better that the gap in my mouth gas not gotten to me. I will have to get an implant as soon as chemo is over. I found out today that my niece is pregnant with a boy! I am so excited! This was just the purpose I needed to take a trip to Hawaii! I was wondering what big life event could bring my out there – nothing better than to celebrate a new life. I am filled with hope that the worst is behind me now. One more big dose of chemo on Monday, and then I'll be on easier street. Can't wait to see Josh in a few weeks!*

November 28:   *Had an AWESOME day! Slept in until around 10 am – had breakfast and ran some errands with Jeff and Maia. Came home and started the turkey around*

2 pm. Did some cleaning and then Maia and I took the dogs on a nice walk. Came home and did some more cleaning which made me feel really good and normal. Started more cooking around 5 and had a great dinner at 6:30. I was able to eat despite my pulled tooth – AND I enjoyed a glass of wine which again made me feel very normal! I have not had a nap all day and am finally in bed at 11:30 pm. I am so grateful for this day and the second chance I have been given to really live the second half of my life. I am feeling so so so so grateful as never before!!!

November 29: *Had a pretty good day – felt good, but low energy. I guess I overdid myself yesterday. I did get out and run some errands, and did some minor cleaning, but spent a lot of time resting. At this point, I really want to get Monday (and next week) over with. I am 1/3 of the way done now, and can't wait until I can say I am half way done, and then just plain DONE! I am trying to decide how to mark the occasion…a tattoo? A major hiking expedition? A marathon? What I really need is a chemical peel, and now an implant! Well, for now I am looking forward to a nice weekend. Must get some Christmas shopping done, at least for Josh, in case I'm not up to it again before he arrives.*

November 30: *Had a horrible nightmare last night – being attacked but couldn't scream. Had a pretty good day, but not such a good night. I am sick of having to worry about every little thing. My temperature has been low – 97.2 – then I got a small scratch on my hand and I* don't have any idea what my white blood cell count is at this point. I feel like the lightest thing might kill me. I hate living this way. Now it is almost 11 pm. I am tired but I am afraid to go to sleep in case I never wake up. I want to live, and really live, not live like this. But if I quit chemo now, I will still be hyper aware, worrying about cancer returning. There is no best answer. I have to see this through — in all its major suckiness.

December 1: Thank God it's December — time is flying! Soon it will be March. Had a rough night last night. Depressed, stressed, and couldn't /wouldn't /didn't sleep/ Slept in and had a pretty decent day. Got some Christmas shopping done anyway. And tomorrow the fun begins again. Nothing to worry about — been there, done that — and this is the last of the "Big" one! I should be thrilled… haha. Feeling less depressed than yesterday — the worst is over and three months goes by fast. Really! March will be here, and I will rebuild my strength and my life better than before. Something to truly look forward to.

December 2: Week 8 it is, and the last of the big chemo dose! I am feeling pretty good tonight — tingly limbs and hot flashes, but nothing horrific. Doc wants me to go in tomorrow for a light white blood boost which doesn't make a lot of sense to me because I am still at 12%. And for three days in a row. Well, I'll just trust that with all that schooling, he knows what he is doing. I'm just happy to not be miserable.

December 3:   *Had a horrific night – I started getting hot flashes. Very sweaty and then my body temp dropped to 96.4. I slept from 12 – 2, 3 – 5, and 8 – 11. Stayed in bed most of the day, just plain tired – but did manage to cook a crock put lamb stew. Went to the Doc at 3:30 for the mild white blood cell boost, ran some errands, and picked Maia up at 5. My bones hurt from the shot, but nothing unbearable or weird. I asked about my low temperature, and the nurse seemed to think that it was an inaccurate reading. Bought an expensive thermometer, but it is still the same tonight. Go figure. Just hoping for a good night sleep and an ok day tomorrow. Jeff will be home!*

December 4:   *A yuck day for sure. Stayed in bed all day feeling like general shit. Had bad gas, bone pain, and all over yuck. However, the chemo fog didn't arrive. I am hoping that today was the worst of it, and I won't have to succumb to the fog tomorrow. Could be, since it has been three weeks since my last chemo. Perhaps this could be the last of the really bad days, and it is all easy street from here! NOT too much to ask! Jeff took are of me all day, and I will be alone tomorrow, so NEED to feel good. The first dose of the new chemo is the next hurdle I have to cross, so I am going to put that worry on hold and enjoy the next two and a half weeks!*

December 5:   *Another sucky day as to be expected. Couldn't make it to the Dr for my injection – must go tomorrow. Was in bed all day, and slept a lot. Slept and ate. Feeling somewhat better now – should be able to go* to the Dr. tomorrow. Hopefully I will also make it to the store – out of food and water.

December 6: Woke up to Maia telling me that Jessee is not feeling well (7:45 am). Maia was able to get her outside to pee, but the poor thing was drooling and breathing hard. I asked Maia to stay home from school in case we needed to take her to the vet. She was able to drink water and sleep. Maia called Jeff, and he said to wait on the vet… I was able to get back to sleep a little bit, then I took Maia down town and went to the Dr. for my injection. Then I made it to the store and back to pick up Maia. Not the best day ever, but typical for a Friday after chemo. Jessee is still not well. She did go out to pee again, but has not eaten, and looks miserable. It will be Jeff's call in the morning what we will do.

December 7: Feeling better and better, but still didn't do much today. Made the mistake of reading too much about Taxol – the next chemo drug I will be on. For some people it is drastically horrific forever! Numb limbs, pain in joints and loss of balance. I will quit if I experience dizziness/loss of balance. For others, it is a breeze – no way to know until I get it. I will try not to worry because I have two weeks here to really enjoy! Jessee is still not feeling well, though she is drinking water and going outside to pee. I hope she will eat tomorrow…I vow to get out of the house and get some exercise!

December 8: Very good day! Got some cleaning done, went to the market, did a lot of cooking, and Jessee ate! We are both feeling so much better. I feel very fragile, and have to keep reminding myself that I am actually fine. There is nothing wrong with me. Jessee and I even went for a little walk. Tomorrow should be a great day. I have a lot of Christmas shopping to do and a To Do list a mile long to complete before Josh gets here in one week. I also want to go for a walk everyday. Hopefully, Jessee will be up for Haney tomorrow. I need to focus on the positive. All is more than well right now. Embrace!

December 9: It is officially week 9! Just 14 to go!! Did some more research this morning on the next round of chemo – seems it is very necessary and most people tolerate it quite well – aside from having their finger and toes to numb (neuropathy). It will be a countdown: 12 – 0 for sure. Most people also loose their eyebrows and lashes after a few weeks and then all hair begins to grow back at about the midway point – that will be exciting for sure! Had a good afternoon – Jessee and I were able to go for a nice walk – we are both getting stronger. Tomorrow I am going Christmas shopping. Yay!

December 10: Productive day! Did some cleaning this morning and then Christmas shopping for two hours – got hungry and tired and had to bail – came home and crashed for a half hour then picked up Maia and we took the dogs to Jensen Beach Causeway – beautiful sunset. Got home and cooked, made cookies. Oh yeah, somewhere in there I went to the Dr. for a white cell boost. I'm sore now and in bed at 10:30. There is still so much to do before Christmas. I'm trying to get as much as I can done before Josh gets here on Monday – at least get his stocking stuffers. So tomorrow is another busy day. Good thing I am feeling up to it for the most part. I wish all I had to worry about was writing my book and getting my body strong. Soon.

December 11: Busy day getting ready for Christmas – can only manage to do about half of what I think needs to be done. I think I must have what is called "chemo brain". I couldn't remember my father's address today – that just doesn't happen (normally). Not even 1 number of it came to me. Got my second shot of neupegen today so my body is tired and achy. It feels like random pins are being stuck into my bones. I should be good tomorrow. I did wander around Target, and Maia and I took the dogs to Haney, but I get tired too fast to accomplish all that I want. We also got pedicures. Yay! I should have a great week ahead. Can't wait to see Josh on Monday – but every day forward is one day closer to the next chemo – YUCK- but also closer to the last one!!

December 12: Another good day in Chemoland! If every day could be like this, I'd be happy, but I have a felling there are going to be a few rough ones up ahead. I have been having hot flashes – not sure if it is just chemo or chemo induced menopause. I haven't had a period since November 1st. Got one step closer to getting Christmas under control. Still so much to do and it doesn't help that I've had a doctor's appointment *every day this week – dentist today. My temperature hit 99 today which I don't like. In bed now at 10:30. I will probably read for another hour – until I can't keep my eyes open. Nights are typically kind of rough. I wake up every two hours in a sweat. I feel hot, then cold – more flashes, but always worse at night. I try not to take my temperature because it can be disturbing (96.4?). A wild ride!*

December 13: *Happy Chemo Day! Got a lot done and enjoyed 2 half glasses of wine this evening which hit me hard. Had to drink two bottles of water to chase it down. My cousin called today. He wanted to wish me well. Apparently he had testicular cancer back before his daughter was born, so he could commiserate with me. He didn't have to do chemo though. Only 6 weeks of radiation – lucky him! Well, I have one more solid week to go! And then the last of the unknowns. Hopefully (a word I use a lot these days) I will be like "most women" and tolerate it well, rather than suffering from deadly allergic reactions and irreversible neuropathy. Just 12 weeks – it will go fast...*

December 14: *All is well here in Chemoland. We went to see Frozen today. It was awesome, but I was so cold during the movie. I wanted to curl up in a fetal position. Next time I go to the movies, I will bring a blanket and ski mask. Also went to Maia's Choir Concert tonight at the high school – totally awesome! And the first time I have been out at night since chemo started. I then enjoyed 2 glasses of wine! Small ones, followed by a* bottle and a half of water. I'm feeling good, but have so much to do tomorrow. I'm looking forward to getting our Christmas tree. Then Josh comes on Monday! Busy, busy!

December 15: I was able to sleep in today to almost 10 am! I've been going, going, going since then! We got our tree and lights up, and I even got a few presents under the tree. I'm finally in bed at 11:00. No nap needed. Will try to rest tomorrow as much as possible – have to take the dogs out for a walk, go to the Dr. at 3 pm for a blood test (hopefully no injections needed) and then pick up Josh at 6:30 in West Palm. I'm sure it will be a busy week with my bro, so rest tomorrow is important. Feeling good!

December 17: Week 10! Great couple of days. Drove to West Palm last night to pick Josh up. Was too tired last night to write – got to bed at midnight. Today we drove to Ft. Pierce to have lunch and go to the beach. Went to the market, came home and I took a much needed nap from 3 – 4 pm. Then we took the dogs for a walk. I dropped Josh off at the gym, picked Maia up, took her to her dermatologist, dropped her off at a soccer game, picked Josh up, and got home around 7 pm. Josh cooked a great healthy dinner, and now it is 11:30 pm... feeling good and tired! Hoping next week won't suck too badly. I may go to the gym tomorrow.

December 18: Lovin' how great I am feeling! It's amazing to look back and know how we all take our health and feeling good for granted. We put our bodies through horrific ordeals, and still they bounce back and don't let us down. I went to the gym today for the first time since I think August. I couldn't do a whole lot, but I did stretch and realized that I am a mess! My body is stiff and tight as a board. Followed that by a treat in the hot tub. I will have to do that more often. Stretch daily and weekly trips to the hot tub. So thrilled to be feeling good!!

December 19: Spent two hours at the beach today with Josh. Very nice and relaxing. Had to take a nap in the afternoon, but otherwise feeling great. I have been taking a vitamin B-complex with biotin every day for the past three days. Will add glutamine three times a day starting Sunday in the hopes of lessening any possible neuropathy from the new chemo – Taxol. Dreading Monday, but feeling hopeful that it actually will treat me better than the AC. Three more days…Josh is going to Miami tomorrow – catching a ride with Jeff in the morning, so I will have the day to myself though Maia comes home early. Last couple of finals for her before Christmas break!

December 20: Josh got a ride with Jeff this morning down to Miami for the night. Jealous. Wish I could enjoy such an endeavor. I took advantage of the situation and rested most of the day. Tried to eat some fattening food! Between Betsy and Josh, I have had nothing but healthy food. It has been great, but I am too thin. Especially in my face. But I swear my hair has started to grow! Still thinking I should shave it completely off now so that I can clearly see the incoming results. So looking forward to a cute short hairdo!

December 21: Josh decided to stay another night in Miami. Probably for the best since Jeff and I rested most of the day, and then went Christmas shopping, and did other regular house stuff. So tomorrow morning I will drive down to West Palm to pick him up. Seahawk game at 4 pm. Then the dreaded week of chemo begins. Every week now. Sounds horrific, but I am feeling better about it. If I have an allergic reaction, I will quit! It is a low dose though, so the side effects should be minimal. Right! Hahaha!! Talking to my friend tomorrow who has been through this particular chemo. In the past few days I have developed ugly dark circles under my eyes. Just 12 weeks to go! Yay!!

December 22: Tomorrow is the Big Day. Well, the other big day after that last big day since the first big day!! I'm feeling pretty good about it - just want it to be over with and to start counting down from 12. I picked up Josh today at the train — other than that the day was pretty uneventful. Still feeling very good. Just hate the dark circles under my eyes. I talked to my friend, and she gave me a crazy list of meds that she took during chemo, and still takes to this day — three years after. She also told me to take a frozen water bottle to hold during chemo to hopefully prevent neuropathy. The Penguin Cap helps women to not lose hair, so why not? Can't hurt.

December 23: Week 11, and my first Taxol. I get to count down backward now to the end! So today was not fun. Josh and I got to the office at 11:15 and waited 30 minutes to see the Doc. Got to the chemo room around 12:15 and all the window seats were taken, so we sat in the back alcove by ourselves. Got my blood work done which came back good, and then the pre med drip around 1 pm. We decided to keep the steroid at 10 mg (half) but to go with their typical dose of Benadryl (50 mg). About half way into the drip, I knew it wasn't going to end well. I felt like I was drowning, and then nauseous. I called for the nurse and Josh held my hand. My body began shaking all over uncontrollably. Two other nurses came over as well...one held my other hand, one massaged my legs, and the other had me do breathing exercises. They were awesome. It took about 30 to 45 minutes for my body to stop shaking. They helped me to the bathroom and waited another 30 minutes before starting the chemo, so by that time it was after 2 pm. I was still feeling like crap, but was ready to get it over with. I felt it as soon as it hit my veins. Tingling in my nose, then my lips, then my chest felt very heavy, and then my arms and legs. I felt better and better as time went on. They increased the drip rate after about an hour, and we finally got out of there around 5 pm. I was still groggy when we got home. Josh made me dinner which I ate in bed, and I have been in bed ever since. It is now 11 pm. So the fun begins.

December 24: It's Christmas Eve! Last night was rough – had hot *flashes/sweats all night – woke up every two hours. I was extremely fatigued all day. I'm not sure if it was a Benadryl hangover, or effects of the chemo. Either way, I was too tired to do anything but stay in bed and eat. At least I didn't feel sick at all. Finally got up at 4 pm to shower and get ready. We had a nice dinner out. I went as Claire. After dinner, we drove through the neighborhood and looked at the lights. We were invited to a party, but I was too tired. We got home at 8 pm and played a nice competitive game of Pictionary. I then took a nice bath and am in bed at 11 pm – after stuffing stockings. Hoping not to be hit by more fatigue tomorrow…this week is an unknown.*

December 26: *Had a great Christmas! Got up at 8 am, did stockings, breakfast, and presents – then took a nap from noon – 2 pm. Had a great dinner that Josh cooked and in bed after midnight. I was too tired to write. Today I woke up with diarrhea and have been in bed all day, and it is Jeff's birthday. I decided I needed to just rest today, so well cook him a special dinner tomorrow. Jeff drove Josh to West Palm to catch his flight home. I have three days before my next treatment, and am starting to get nervous. Some people have an allergic reaction during the second dose. I think it's odd that I felt tingling in my nose and lips and chest and can't find that anywhere as a side effect during an infusion. Plus, the Benadryl dose will be less- which is good unless something goes wrong.*

December 27:   *I finally feel like I can start to make a life plan for the next 3 months! If all goes well on Monday, which it will, I am going to start taking a yoga and/or Pilates class and I'd like to take the photography class at Elliot museum now that I have a nice shiny new red camera to play with. I may even be able to get some writing done as long as the neuropathy stays away. I just took a hot bath and now feel some tingling in my right (writing) hand. But mostly I feel good – more tired than what should be normal, but not yucky like with the AC chemo. I am not even dreading Monday – just a little nervous about it as any normal person would be. Diarrhea is gone, and all is well.*

December 29:   *So all of my facial hair is gone except my eyebrows and lashes, and my face is like a baby's butt! So soft. I still have upper arm and leg hair – no under arm or pubes. Josh shaved my head on Christmas – it looks much better than it did with just scraggly 1 inch hairs. I can't wait to see fuzz! Tomorrow is the dreaded chemo day – had a good weekend, and not such a bad week, but starting to get nervous again about the infusion – especially with the lowered dose of steroids and Benadryl. Good God. Why does treatment have to be potentially life threatening? On the bright side – if all goes well, I can start planning my life for the next few months!*

December 30:   *What a day! Went to the Dr. fully expecting to get chemo…told him about my immediate reaction last week ie. Tingling nose, numb lips, heave/tingling* chest and legs, and he seemed to think that I was having a serious allergic reaction and without the aid of Benadryl could be life threatening. He basically gave me three options. Go ahead with Taxol and if I get a reaction (likely), I would be pumped with more Benadryl. Um...NO! Or opt out of chemo altogether, or try a different Taxane like Abraxane...not likely covered by insurance. We left saying I would think about it, and in the meantime, he would order the Abraxane and see if it is covered by my insurance. So many mixed feelings today, but all in all – happy to be chemo free!

January 1: Had a great New Year's Eve with the neighbors. So happy so say goodbye to 2013! 2014 is here and I am so excited about all of the things I want to do. I have decided to opt out o the final chemo. I feel in my heart/gut, that it would do more harm than good, so I will be moving on to radiation. I don't see the Doc until the 13th so I don't know the exact plan yet, but tomorrow I see the surgeon and I am going to try out a yoga class. I also need to get my diet in order and do away with cigarettes for good by Monday! Can't wait to get back to life and also to grow some hair! I am feeling great about the year to come!!

January 2: I felt like such a normal person today, despite being bald. I saw my surgeon this morning – he said my boobs look great! Went shopping, ate an awesomely healthy lunch of salmon and spinach, Maia and I took the dogs to Haney, and then we went to the gym!! My first real day back. I took a yoga class – it was good. Just easy enough for me. Will probably get bored of it soon, but it is great way for me to get back into working out. I am stiff and sore all over. Then Maia and I made healthy smoothies before she took off to meet her friends, and I made another healthy meal- whole wheat pasta with a turkey squash sauce. I enjoyed it! Just got out of a nice hot bath and am in bed at 10 pm. Will read for an hour.

January 7: I see it's been almost a week since I've been here! I guess that means that for the most part, life is back to normal – but not really. There isn't a day (or probably an hour) that goes by that I don't think about cancer and possible death. I think my hair is growing! Very slowly, but yeah. I've also make serious dietary changes. No simple carbs – using whole wheat and veggie oriented pastas and drinking smoothies with berries and yogurt – trying to emulate the high vitamin B17 diet of the indigenous cultures that are 100% cancer free. Getting raw nuts in the US is a problem, but the berries, whole wheat and spinach will do for now.

January 9: I am scared. That's a fact. If you ask anyone, they would say I have a positive attitude, and am happy...I don't want to die. I don't want to die now. I know I will die some day, but I am scared of death, and I don't want it to come early for me. I don't want to leave Maia motherless. I don't want to leave Jeff partnerless. I don't want to leave a whole in the lives of my sister, brother, mother, family...I could die. I know it. I am not ready. I am afraid. It *never goes away – the fear. I feel it hit my veins through my arms, cold hard ugly fear. I have not wanted to write about it, but it is there. I want to live. I don't want to exist in fear. I want to really live, without the fear. I want to not be afraid of death. I don't want it to come until I am ready.*

January 13: *And so the fun resumes in a week. Saw Dr. Dread today and apparently Abraxane was approved – not what I was expecting. I have been living a normal life these past few weeks and my hair is even growing. I was both happy and devastated at the news that I will be continuing chemo starting next week. All the research points to the benefits of a Taxane for triple negative breast cancer. It's a no brainer – just not easy to digest from here – 3 weeks out of chemo. It is better than recurrence though, which is associated with much more certain death. Chemo through March. Can do!*

January 14: *So I am resigned to the fact that I will resume chemo on Monday. I guess I am supposed to think that that is a good thing. It's hard since I don't have active cancer, to really embrace it. I want to do all I can to make sure, and to have peace of mind that I have done all I can to prevent a recurrence. I do have positive thoughts about Abraxane, and that it will not be horrible. Hard to erase the memory of my Benadryl/Taxol experience but soon it will. I have to start living like I am living, and not like I am going to be dead soon or already am. Oh, the dark thoughts. Oh, the fear of death. LIVE, LIVE, LIVE. It's all* *temporary anyway. Right?*

January 15:   *So I guess I didn't take my own advice yet from what I wrote yesterday. Got up today around 9:30 and began researching cancer – I was looking at P53 and KI67 expression and relative chemo resistance – the studies seem to be contradictory but all point to the effectiveness of Taxanes ie Taxol, Taxotere, Abraxane – which I should point out that I specifically requested thinking that my insurance would never cover it...Anyway, point being that I stress myself out and am counter productive. I am getting chemo – Abraxane – on Monday – I've agreed to it and I think I should do it, but I continue to stress over it and research when it is a given. I need to stop the MADNESS!!*

January 16:   *OK – so I finally remember what it is like to live! Went to the gym today – could only run a 12 minute mile – but it felt great! Spent some time learning photography, did some cleaning and shopping, and only thought about cancer once every two hours!! Three more days until I am back to chemo. Need to make the most of these days, but also the ones to come. What I need to do REALLY, is get back to my writing. I have a book that needs revising and it is so close to being finished. I can easily do that over the next 11 weeks. The gym also needs to be a regular part of my day/week. I felt so good today!*

January 17:   *So...I have about 1/6 of an inch of fuzz on my head,* *my eyebrows and lashes are still there, but thinned. I had to shave my legs today, still have arm hair, no pubic or under arm hair though. That's the hair update! Didn't really have a good day. Depression is here already. Wasn't as productive as I would like to be – worked some on my book. The day went by too quickly – researched colleges for Maia – got excited about that but generally I'm feeling very down. Didn't make any of the phone calls that I had set out to make. I hate wasting days.*

January 18: *Count down to Chemo: 48 hours! What I have is: triple negative, high grade (3), KI67 100%, P53 100%, breast cancer. Seems like a death sentence! But I refuse to live like I am dying. Won't anymore! Gonna enjoy the shit out of life! Just found out that my mother may have a recurring tumor. She had breast cancer about 10 years ago – estrogen positive – so not the same as mine. Abnormal mammo – could be nothing. Also just found out that her mother died of breast cancer. All this time, I thought she died of lung cancer. Well, in the end she did, but only because she had three lumps removed from her breast on three separate occasions, on three consecutive years with no further treatment that spread to her lungs.*

January 20: *Another big hurdle crossed! Got my 1st round of Abraxane this afternoon. Was pretty depressed all morning, but took the dogs out with Maia which was good for the exercise and to take my mind off things. Got to treatment at 2 pm, in the chair by 2:30 ish, blood work drawn – wait for the chemo to mix – got* pre-meds (including steroids which took me by surprise). By the time I got the chemo it was around 4 pm! That part was the quickest. No reactions, just fidgety from the steroid. Feel tired tonight more than usual, and gassy but not bad. Got pizza and watched a movie. There was a 68 year old woman next to me getting the same chemo. She said it was her favorite kind (lol). She has inoperable pancreatic cancer, and not long to live. There was also a girl a little younger than Maia getting treatment. I should feel blessed.

January 21: Feeling pretty good today. I even went to the gym and walked the dogs. I was tired and needed to rest several times, but this chemo is sooo much easier than the first two – especially AC. I can't believe it's already January and I still have al least 10 more weeks to go. It may be more if they do three weeks on then one week off. Not sure yet. As long as I can function, I guess its ok. Just need to worry about not getting sick, especially with winter here. I am going to start getting Runs Like the Wind ready for publishing. I'm feeling optimistic that this week will not be so bad. No signs of neuropathy!

January 23: I have been working on my book these past two days. I am now excited to get it out there! I am about halfway through editing, and did all the formatting which was the big job – though I'll probably have to go back through it. Just need to get Jeff to do the cover. I have felt pretty good all week – I just get tired easily- like bone tired, and have to rest. I don't really nap – like go to sleep – but some times I need an entire hour to lie down. My hair is really blooming, and I am praying that I don't lose it. 10 weeks sounds so short, but yet so long!

January 27:   I have lost track of what week I am on – way off schedule now, but I do know that I had drip #3 today with 9 to go. How I hate sitting in the Big Chair, but in reality, it wasn't so bad. Jeff was with me and I brought a pack of frozen peas to put on my head under my hat. The trick is supposed to be that if your hands, fingers, and toes are at a cold enough temperature you won't get neuropathy or lose your hair. So I hold a frozen water bottle, and apply the pea pack during infusion. So far so good. My hair is long enough that you can actually see it from across the room! It is like a 5 O'clock shadow. I want to keep it! It looks brown to me but it is very soft and fine. I have been conditioning it every other day! That is actually the cheerier side of my day – here is the darker side. I woke up in the middle of the night with a pain/ache in my lower abdomen. I did an internet search and was convinced that I have ovarian cancer. Later, I decided it was probably just gas – which my Doc agreed with. Last week I was sure I had a new lump in my breast and that my mole is cancerous. The week before that I had a headache, and was convinced that I have brain cancer. I am trying to remind myself that I am fine! I HAD cancer, and chemo sucks, but I am going to be fine. It is ok to feel good! It is ok to be healthy! I am cancer free!! I think this is week 15 – and 12 to go- so past the halfway point (if I don't count rads).

February 2:   *Had a great birthday weekend! Connie arrived on Friday. Saturday was my 47th birthday and we went to Jupiter to the Blowing Rock Preserve. Maia and I took our cameras and we had a nice time on the beach. Connie and I went in for a dip. We came home and Jeff and I napped while Connie and Maia took the dogs out. Then we went out for dinner. It was a great day, and I felt great. Connie and I stayed up way too late and drank way too much wine! It feels good to feel normal! Today Jeff bought a car and the Seahawks won the Super bowl! Another great day. My hair is still growing and tomorrow I go to chemo and Connie goes home. Looking forward to taking my photography class and getting my book done.*

February 3:   *Number 9 done! 8 to go... WBC count is at the low end of normal. I need to make it through the week without getting sick. No chemo next week – yay! But will see the Doc on Monday and get blood re-checked – if it drops, which I'm thinking it will, I will get a boost. There was a young woman next to me today, 32 – and it was her very first chemo day. It felt good to offer some advice and to get to feel good that I am done with that chemo (AC), and am over the hump, but I felt bad for what she is going to go through over the next two months. I hope I will get to see her again next chemo day to find out how she managed. I am hoping it will be easier for her. I forgot to mention that I lost my implant crown this weekend. I think I swallowed it the night before my birthday. Friday it had fallen out (again) and I glued it back in, but* while I was eating breakfast the next morning, my birthday breakfast, I noticed it was gone. Called the dentist today. It will cost $900 to replace. Oh, shit!!

February 6: All is well. I've been tired the past few days, but still well enough to shop, walk the dogs, cook and do some cleaning. Went to the dentist today, but didn't realize they need to remove the stump to do an impression for my crown, which would have meant going into my gums – and blood. I wouldn't let them do it...afraid my WBC counts are too low right now, so I will have to get a boost on Monday/Tuesday and have it done next Thursday. No chemo next week – Yay! Was looking forward to having a productive week, but looks like I will be at the doctor or dentist every day. Well, I do have tomorrow! Very tired tonight. Hoping for a great night sleep. Must get up at 7:45 to take Maia to school.

February 9: No chemo tomorrow! And just 11 weeks to go with 8 more infusions and then on to radiation. It will be one year round trip. Uneventful weekend, though Jeff and I did go fishing this evening for about an hour. I'm still tired more than usual for a Sunday, but have one whole week to recoup despite all the trips to the doctor and dentist. Cut myself twice this weekend – always worries me when I know my WBC count is low. Hoping for a boost tomorrow. Gonna work on my book in the morning, and off to the doctor at 2:15.

February 14: All is well. Jeff and I had a nice Valentine's day. We *made a lot of pupu's for dinner and made love. It had been a while so we were both nervous. Maybe not the best word to describe it, but all in all we need to get back in to that groove! Had a scary mammogram this week which I haven't written about – found a lump in my left breast after months of not giving myself a breast exam. Doc agreed that it felt suspicious though he said it was probably just a breast abnormality. Who gets cancer in the other breast while on chemo? Well, after searching the internet, I would say just about no one!! Even the radiologist was surprised that I was there getting a mammo on the unaffected breast. Well, I don't regret doing it. Doc had his office assistant call that same afternoon after the results were in to let me know that everything is fine! That was very sweet. I wish this week off of chemo had been more productive I did finish editing Runs Like the Wind and found a potential translator for the Navajo parts, but didn't finish the cover page which I had hoped to do. 8 more treatments to go. 3 weeks on, one off, 3 weeks on, one off, then just two weeks on – then I don't know how many off before radiation.*

February 17: *Happy Chemo Day! Everything went smoothly today. Just felt a little yucky this evening. Couldn't nap because of the steroid. Nurse N said she would drop the steroid down to 4 mg next week (down from 10). Maybe I will feel much better and hopefully won't get nauseous! Poor girl next to me today had just come from having her port put in and was nauseated from the anesthetic. She threw up twice and I* *thought I might join her. I can't imagine getting chemo (Red Devil) right after port surgery. I hope they had a good reason for doing that to her. Saw Janet – the girl from last time. She said the last two weeks were pretty rough for her. I was not sitting near her, though, so I didn't get to hear what happened. I hope her Dr. adjusted it for her and the next two weeks won't be so bad. Maybe we can chat more next time…in two weeks. My WBC count is at 6.2%. I hope it doesn't drop too much during week 3 of this round. 2 two more, then a week off – get my implant back during my week off, and only 5 more to go after all that!!!*

February 20: *So I have been a little depressed the past couple of weeks. Couldn't sleep Monday night as usual because of the steroids so Tuesday was a waste. Woke up at 7 am on Wednesday feeling very good and thought I would have a great productive day, but my computer was broken – spent most of the day trying to fix it but couldn't, and then the depression set in. Woke up late today with major bone aches all over and a general very tired feeling. I am just so over this. I want my effking life back! Then I'm scared of not being on chemo because my body is vulnerable. I can't win! Have to keep reminding myself that MOST women do not EVER have a recurrence. There is no real reason to think I will…*

February 23: *Back to chemo tomorrow. Not as depressing as last Sunday with the week off. Just want it over with. The bone pain has tapered off but I don't think I will* *be able to do the photography class on Thursdays. Bummer for now- added to a lot of other bummers! My hair is holding on. Not really growing so much, but not falling out! It is a covering and I have gone to not wearing a head covering at home. It is no longer disturbing to Maia or Jeff or me. After tomorrow, I will be half way through Abraxane!! Yay!! Only six to do. No neuropathy. Still on the fence about radiation. Will wait to make the decision after discussing with the doctor.*

February 24: *Six to go! They didn't reduce my steroid – oh, well. Took a hot bath, hoping to sleep tonight. This morning I started having some tingling in my right index finger. Not bad enough to call it neuropathy. Got diarrhea tonight after a Chinese food dinner. Having hot flashes now. I'm hoping I won't be in pain this week and will able to make it to the photography class on Thursday morning. I was going to cancel but got an email reminder today and I feel bad not going. Besides, I really want to go! My computer is still not working. I don't think it came with back up software so we can't wipe it out. Hoping Jeff will work his magic soon and make it come back to life!*

March 2: *Happy Birthday to Auntie Connie! Tomorrow is chemo day #7. Only 5 to go – one week off, then 3 – then a week off, then the last 2!! Had a good week – was able to go to my photography class on Thursday – really enjoyed it, and learned a lot. Was sooo, sooo, tired after. Slept from 2 – 4 pm and Maia took the* dogs out alone. Got joint/muscle pain that night which lasted through yesterday (Saturday). Tingling still in right finger tips. Nothing too bad. Advil for the pain works fine. Got my computer working today!! Not dreading tomorrow too much.

March 8: I am missing Connie's big 70ᵗʰ birthday bash tonight. She was planning it a year ago when she visited and I promised to be there but I'm not there. I'm here. I'm sure she understands... LOL!! Had a pretty good week. Loving my photography class on Thursdays though it wipes me out after. No chemo next week – yay! Then only 5 to go! Double yay!! Hoping to get together with Aaron and Jonelle next weekend.

March 17: Had last week chemo free! Felt quite productive though get tired often. Today is #8 – only 4 to go after that! Had a good weekend – went to dinner with Aaron and Jonelle. Drank too much and had a very lazy Sunday, but it was good to get out and see people. I'm loving my photography class on Thursdays, but am sooo tired by the end. Only 6 more weeks of this, then 6 more of radiation. The end is in sight! Then of course, I have to worry about a recurrence which could kill me. Lovely. But looking forward to a healthy productive year ahead. Hair is still growing – about an inch now, but too thin in front for me to feel comfortable going hatless. I think I will debut my hair right when chemo is done. It should be just long enough by then.

March 24: Last week, the steroid was lowered from 10 mg to 5.

No diarrhea on Monday – but more tired than usual all week – perhaps not related to the steroid and more because I am getting to the end. Got my computer fixed on Tuesday and Thursday is the last photo class for now. Friday the termite man came. Had dinner last night with Kim, Chuck, Aaron and Jonelle. Great to see everyone. Kim and Chuck drive back to LA with their furniture today. I'm going for #9 in a few hours. Only 3 to go after today! My hair has thinned out a lot – kind of depressing. Perhaps I will go back to the peas today. I want hair! Jeff is much happier after his promotion 2 weeks ago, so things are getting done. Life feels a little livelier!

March 31: *So last week sucked until about Friday when I started feeling normal again. Today I had #10! Yay!! Yay for April starting tomorrow! I have next week off so should be good and productive and then only 2 more to go. I can't believe the end of chemo is finally in sight!! It's been a long six months. Debby comes tomorrow, so I plan on resting all day so that I can cook dinner and be sociable when she's here. Hoping I can sleep tonight, but I'm not counting on it. I am so tired, but either the chemo or the steroid, or the combo doesn't like sleep. Jeff made me a nice salmon dinner, and the three of us watched "Mud". Good movie. I feel ok, not so great, not terrible. Headache and hot flashes. ALMOST DONE!!*

April 14: *We are on our way! Just one more to go! I had a slower recovery after the last set of three. Was very sluggish until Friday and didn't fell good until*

Tuesday of my off week. Was semi pretty productive after that. Got *Runs Like the Wind* completely edited and am working on the cover page. Hoping I can finish it over the next two weeks. Feeling pretty crappy today after chemo. Headache, heart palpitations, tired, and just basically off. A little better now after dinner, a movie and a cool bath. Hot flashes have kicked in again. Hoping for a good night sleep – ha ha! I will be officially done with chemo in one week from today! Too bad I'll feel too shitty to celebrate!

April 15:   I've decided to keep a daily log this week because I have been a little light headed lately and I want to narrow down the exact times/cause – don't want an MRI. Of course brain cancer is in the back of my mind – or mostly in the front of my mind which may be part of the cause – anxiety. A couple of weeks ago, I had a strange headache in the back of my head, and that got me worried, and then the headache went away after two days, and I felt light headed. Dizzy isn't exactly the right word for it. It happens when I am lying down or sitting back and I feel better if I get up and walk. It's more like my head is swimming. I didn't get my CBC yesterday, but I have been taking 2 iron pills per day to help with my perpetual low RBC count. I slept off and on last night (my insomnia night) for a total of 7 ½ hours – not bad! Still tired, but not horrible and I do feel somewhat anxious. But not dizzy. This never happens when I'm walking. So I think that's a good thing. My ear also feels stuffy and two weeks ago it ached – right ear,

then left. So maybe it is inner ear related from chemo.
When I was on Adriamycin I had vertigo when
turning from left to right in bed, but this is different.
It happens when I'm flat on my back. I am going to
work on relaxation this week, and hope it's gone by
Monday. If not, I will have to tell the Doc, which
almost certainly means the dreaded MRI. I don't
know which I fear most – the actual MRI or the
results.

April 16: Well, I called the nurse yesterday because I had a dull
ache in my heart after the infusion on Monday
accompanied by heart flip flops. – forgot to write
about that yesterday because I was all consumed
with the dizziness which doesn't seem to be a factor
right now. The nurse spoke to the Dr and told me to
see a cardiologist ASAP. Yay me!! But to go through
my regular physician. She is on vacation, so I have an
appointment with her in two weeks. I wanted to see
her anyway for menopause related sexual problems.
So now I am 90% sure that I am going to opt out of
the final chemo treatment. Going to talk to nurse N
today to get her opinion, and then she can pass the
info on to the Doc. But I think I am done –
baked…cooked…toxined out!

April 17: Talked to nurse N yesterday, and she strongly
suggested that I go to the ER – two weeks would be
too long to see someone about my heart. After 6 long
hours, an EKG, a chest x-ray, a CT scan, and
countless blood tests, I was told that my heart was
strong, but the EKG showed abnormal behavior,

most likely due to chemo induced arrhythmia. The doctor there advised that I do no have any more chemo, and said he would send a follow up note to my oncologist. So it's official – NO MORE CHEMO!!! It feels very anticlimactic because I didn't finish, but I know my body can't take anymore. I got home at 10:30 last night, had a bath, and went to bed. I've been in bed all day, resting, but finally got up at 4 pm and took the dogs out with Maia. I am going to drive her to a friend's house soon. The house is a wreck. I hope I feel better/get some energy tomorrow.

April 18: Well, no luck on having energy today! But, feeling somewhat better. Friday is the new Tuesday. But none of that matters because it is the last Friday I will ever feel this bad! Every day from here is a better day, and I vow to do something with these days!

April 20: Well, I am still feeling a little "off". Not really sure how to describe it. It started about 4 infusions ago. Just not quite right – but every day I feel better, and every morning I am surprised, and happy to be alive. Today was a great Easter Sunday. We took the boat out, dyed eggs, had a nice ham dinner, and watched the sunset. I didn't nap at all, but did rest a couple of times. I am so relieved that I am not having chemo tomorrow as originally planned. I do see the Doc though. Hopefully to talk about radiation. Just had a nice bath, and am feeling very tired and relaxed. Can't wait for tomorrow and am even better day! I am starting to plan our Key Largo vacation!

April 22:   I am really done with chemo! It's kind of hard for me to believe – it's been a way of life for 6 long months. I can't believe it's really over! Saw the Doc yesterday – he was fine with me skipping the last one. Now on to radiation in a couple of weeks – an adventure of another color. There is no way it will be as brutal as chemo. I'm feeling better and better everyday. Next week should be a very good one. Doc said I am probably not ready for a gym workout but I can go ahead with yoga. I think that is a great place to start. Looking forward to getting my life back!!!

April 28:   I am now 2 weeks out of chemo. Can't believe – looking back – that I didn't write about me thinking I had brain cancer. Maybe it was just too scary. Had ringing in my ears, dizziness, stuffy ears, and muffling. More than likely another chemo side effect. Ototoxicity and Tinnitus are caused by chemo and I do feel better ever day. Went to the Look Good, Feel Better program today. Did my makeup and came home with a new wig – Samantha! It was really fun. One step closer to book publishing, and feeling better every day!

May 12:   I am 4 weeks out of chemo and still very much feeling the aftermath. I get dizzy when I am tired, don't eat, or concentrate too long at the computer. Still, rarely but sometimes have an earache in my right ear. Still have to nap everyday, and still feel tired. I think I am better every day, but I am frustrated that I still feel this tired after a month. On the positive side, I published my book on May 7th! Feels good, but hoping it doesn't get buried in Amazon. Had a great Mother's Day – took the boat out to the sandbar and lunch in Manatee Cove. Maia got me an adorable, outstanding white sun dress which I have been wanting for years!! Jeff got me my favorite perfume and a seafood fest dinner. I met with the radiation oncologist last week – supposed to start next Monday. I DON'T WANT TO! I so feel that my body has had enough torture/damage, and I am not recovered from chemo but here we go again… On a very sad note, Kathryn's niece, only 25, was diagnosed with breast cancer last week. I pray she doesn't have to do chemo. 25 is too young to have to deal with this shit. And last, but not least, I went to FT Lauderdale last Thursday for Jeff's company party and stayed the night at the Sheraton next door. We had a great time. Just can't believe he does that commute every single morning and night.

May 16: Had the best day ever in such a long time. Went to Pilates this morning, had good energy the rest of the day. Not sure if it was a coincidence or the exercise, but I felt really good – almost normal. Went to Maia's spring choir concert tonight, then we went out for sushi which I had been craving since forbidden to eat it since last October. It is now almost midnight and I haven't napped all day! I imagine I will sleep in tomorrow, but I feel good. My port has started aching off and on, though. It is due for a flush so maybe that is why. I think I will have it removed soon.

May 22:   *I am disappointed in myself because I don't write about the horrors. Every week or so for the last 8 months I have been convinced that I am dying of something. Cancer (duh), but so many that I don't even remember. Most recently, it was my port. It began hurting and I was sure I had a blood clot that would get to my lungs/heart and I would die. I finally got a logical explanation that it was because I had to keep my arms up for 35 minutes twice in one week for radiation and it strained the underlying muscle. Now the latest...I had a dream that Betsy had breast cancer – there was an image of her breast on a computer screen and it obviously had a huge lump. The doctor said "the cancer is back". I woke up just as the words were being spoken – it sounded like words in my ear. It also sounded like the voice that I link to my guardian angel who once said – 15 years ago- "check your baby" – the night that I found Maia tangled in her sheets and felt that that voice saved her life. I live in fear. I don't want to! That voice and those words have haunted me for three days now. I will keep going.*

May 31:   *Well, I am still my worst enemy. I've been doing great going to Pilates, yoga, but developed high blood pressure – 150/100 at worst. Was checking it every day – best 124/95. Always around 95. Thought I would go to the ER today because my arms and fingers went numb. I decided to put mind over matter. Jeff and I went walking on the beach, had a picnic and then checked back in for blood pressure* which had dropped to 124/84! Yay! Time to stop living in fear...

June 1:

I went out without my headscarf for the first time today! With Jeff's approval, but without Maia's – she said I look like a baby penguin. Ha ha!! At least I am cute!! Not really... Did a lot of cleaning today. Took the power pressure washer to the patio, and then bought some new plants. Feeling good. Checked my blood pressure this afternoon – still high at 134/89. Not horrible. Just took a bath and a Bayer aspirin.

June 9:

Blood pressure is still high – which is causing anxiety, which came first, the chicken or the egg? That is a good question here. At radiation today it was 150/114 – later on my own it was 136/90. Not happy with that. One day, I hope to wake up with no stress. I am sad that almost 2 months post chemo I am still having such issues. On the bright side, my hair has really come in! I no longer wear hats/bandanas/anything, and I won't ever again! Maia's friends still haven't seen me so I'm a little nervous about that – but it is what it is. I have been going to the gym twice a week – love the Pilates, but not so fond of the yoga there (I prefer the one at the Cancer Center). Too much up and down! I am seeing my oncologist on Thursday in PSL because my port has been hurting still, and no one can offer a reasonable explanation, so of course, I fear the worst. I just had a bath and I bet if I took my blood pressure right now it would make me happy, but I think I have given myself a white coat and there is no way to give me a good reading. I will have to find a way to trick myself!

June 12:   Saw the Doc today. I pushed up my appointment that was scheduled for Monday because of the port issue and high blood pressure. I asked the nurse not to take by blood pressure due to white coat silliness, and she agreed to take it later and then came back and took it right away "out of curiosity" she said. It was 150/86. I was relieved. The Doc didn't think any thing was seriously wrong with my port, so I am going to see my surgeon tomorrow about it. My CBC came back good, but they also took blood for a tumor marker test. Routine, but terrifying. I hope I don't hear from them tomorrow.

June 16:   I am getting my port out tomorrow! I saw Dr. K – not L, and he said if it hurts, it's time for it to go! Yay! I wish it were L, though taking it out because apparently K insists on putting you under and L will do it with just a local anesthetic in the office. It's much more of an ordeal this way, and I hate going under, but it will be OUT! No dreaded call about tumor markers, and more than halfway through radiation. Maybe now I can stop stressing – ha ha. Not likely, but maybe my blood pressure will go back to normal. That would be nice. Going to The Keys in two weeks!! Can't wait!!!

June 21:   I am officially de-ported! Surgery was fine – waited a long time, but it only took 15 minutes. I was *allowed to be awake through it and it was a breeze. I was in some pain the first couple of days, especially after radiation because I have to hold my arms over my head, but so glad it is gone!! I have 10 more radiation treatments to go. Taking a week off when we go to the Keys and then only 5 more. I am feeling a little fatigued – take a nap in the afternoon and my breast is sunburned, but all in all, nothing to complain about. Yay! No issues!!!*

July 7:   *Had a blast in The Keys – 3 days went way too fast. But we managed to pack it in – went sailing, kayaking, snorkeling, and on a nice sunset cruise. Came home tired but feeling good. We've been working on putting in our new bamboo flooring. My breast sunburn in getting better, but I go back to radiation today – only four more to go! Yay! Tomorrow I will go back to Pilates and get in a regular gum schedule, and writing time. I still get worn out easily, but after this week, my energy level can only improve. Back to life!! Looking for a job, getting a fence put in, finishing the floor, and writing my book. Maia got her driver's license!! Sweet 16!! WOO HOO!!*

July 14:   *I am officially done with radiation which also means done with cancer treatment!!! Funny how it ends with no real BANG. It's just over. We have decided to go to New York for Christmas – super excited about that. Still tired every day, but my hair is growing very thick. It isn't very long, maybe one inch at the thickest point, and a weird color. Baby poop green is how I describe it. I have been putting sun-in in for the past two days. Looking a little blonder!!*

August 1: *Three weeks out of radiation now. Feeling a lot more energy and skin has healed. But still not out of Cancer Hell. Saw the Doc on Monday — got the dreaded call on Wednesday that my CEA tumor marker blood test was high. I thought after Tuesday that I would be free and clear from such calls. So Wednesday was a surprise. Not horribly elevated — 4.6. Nurse N said that for a smoker, or even former smoker that could be normal, but apparently they haven't been doing this test all along, so they have nothing to compare it to except for post surgery when it was 6. Got another call from them today that they want to do anther test. Oh joy, and a PET scan in September.*

August 24: *I am now 6 weeks post radiation and 4 months post chemo. Feeling more normal every day. The CEA retake was still high, but in the normal range. So no alarm bells were set off. A couple of weeks ago I started having joint pain — fingers and toes (maybe that's neuropathy), but also in elbows, and shoulders. I thought I had bone cancer, but it is now getting better. I'm still stiff in the morning, but it goes away mostly after abut a half hour. My hair is getting longer — about 2 inches, and it is also getting quite curly! It's now blonde. Maia went back to school, so I now have a golden opportunity to pore myself into writing!!*

September 17: Time is flying by. I can't believe it has been 5 months since the end of chemo and 2 since radiation. My hair is looking pretty ridiculous – may be time for my first hair cut. Just realized that a year ago tomorrow was the lumpectomy. Wow! Today I had a chest x-ray and mammogram – both ordered by L. Funny thing is that the radiologist and doctor that read the mammo questioned if I really had had breast cancer! What? As if I could make that shit up! Apparently, Dr. L did such a great job that there is no scar tissue or "markers" left behind. Not sure what that means, but I will have to tell him!

September 26: Mamma and chest x-ray came back clean. Next is the PET scan on Monday. Everyone says I have nothing to worry about, but I wouldn't be getting one if there were really nothing to worry about! And my leg has been hurting, so of course I am worried about bone cancer. It's my knee area that hurts, so probably nothing to worry about, but f course I will. The PET scan itself won't be so bad – it will be the following Monday when I see the Doc for the results. I do not know how I am going to get through that appointment! I fly to San Diego two days after for B's 50th birthday, so it better come back clean!

October 5: Had the PET scan last Monday. When I was leaving, the tech said, "so I guess I will never see you again". So I felt really good about how it had gone. Obviously he sees the screen while it's happening. It was much easier this time around compared to one year ago. But then on Thursday, the back of my head started to hurt, so again, I worried about bone cancer – might have been stress. I get the official results tomorrow, and I fly to San Diego on Wednesday. Hoping to not have a panic attack!

October 7:   PET scan came back good – though he had to scare me first by telling me there was some activity in my right breast. Then he said probably due to scar tissue forming after radiation. It is getting harder and feels bigger! I was hoping to be elated, but instead I have a big fat stress headache! Going to San Diego tomorrow!! Hopefully that will take care of the stress. I may have to splurge on a massage. No more doctors for 3 months. Maybe I can get back to normal finally. My hair looks like it might have a style – a funky curly one.

October 24:   San Diego was great! Good to see Betsy, Josh, and meet his girlfriend, and see Kenya. Got a call while I was there form the oncologist's office. I freaked when I saw the phone number because I had had the tumor marker test done on Monday – however, it was just Nurse N calling to ask if I still needed the Chantix prescription. Hard to believe that one year ago, I was just starting chemo. My hair was just starting to fall out. So glad that year is over. It's been six months since chemo. Time is flying where it stood still last year.

CHEMOLAND

www.ingramcontent.com/pod-product-compliance
Lightning Source LLC
Chambersburg PA
CBHW060515290526
45791CB00001B/396